Enduring Negativity

Modern French Identities

Edited by Peter Collier

Volume 96

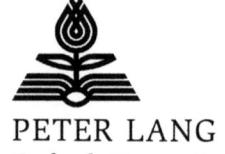

PETER LANG
Oxford · Bern · Berlin · Bruxelles · Frankfurt am Main · New York · Wien

Charlotte Baker

Enduring Negativity

Representations of Albinism in
the Novels of Didier Destremau,
Patrick Grainville and
Williams Sassine

PETER LANG
Oxford · Bern · Berlin · Bruxelles · Frankfurt am Main · New York · Wien

Bibliographic information published by Die Deutsche Nationalbibliothek
Die Deutsche Nationalbibliothek lists this publication in the Deutsche
Nationalbibliografie; detailed bibliographic data is available on the
Internet at http://dnb.d-nb.de.

A catalogue record for this book is available from the British Library.

Library of Congress Cataloging-in-Publication Data:

Baker, Charlotte, 1976-
  Enduring negativity : representations of albinism in the novels of
Didier Destremau, Patrick Grainville and Williams Sassine / Charlotte
Baker.
       p. cm. -- (Modern French identities ; 96)
  Includes bibliographical references and index.
  ISBN 978-3-0343-0179-4 (alk. paper)
  1. French fiction--20th century--History and criticism. 2. Albinos
and albinism in literature. 3. Destremau, Didier, 1937---Criticism and
interpretation. 4. Grainville, Patrick, 1947---Criticism and
interpretation. 5. Sassine, Williams, 1944---Criticism and
interpretation. I. Title.
  PQ673.B35 2011
  843'.914093561--dc22
                                        2011004206

ISSN 1422-9005
ISBN 978-3-0343-0179-4

© Peter Lang AG, International Academic Publishers, Bern 2011
Hochfeldstrasse 32, CH-3012 Bern, Switzerland
info@peterlang.com, www.peterlang.com, www.peterlang.net

All rights reserved.
All parts of this publication are protected by copyright.
Any utilisation outside the strict limits of the copyright law, without
the permission of the publisher, is forbidden and liable to prosecution.
This applies in particular to reproductions, translations, microfilming,
and storage and processing in electronic retrieval systems.

Printed in Germany

Contents

Acknowledgements — vii
Introduction — 1

CHAPTER 1
The Albino Body — 23
    Chromatic Ambivalence — 25
    A Deficient Body — 36
    Disability — 41
    The Transforming Body — 47
    Freakery — 50

CHAPTER 2
Myth and Stereotype — 57
    The Stereotypes of Albinism — 58
    Alternative Explanations — 65
    The Stigma of Albinism — 70
    Myths Surrounding Albinism — 72
    Sacrifice — 77

CHAPTER 3
Inclusion and Exclusion — 87
    Forms of Exclusion — 88
    Social Exile — 93
    The 'Passing' Albino — 95
    A Mark of Belonging — 98
    The Cost of Inclusion — 103

CHAPTER 4
Inhabiting the Margins 113
- Borders, Boundaries and Divisions 114
- The Threat of the Ambiguous 116
- Geographical Margins 122
- Multiple Centres, Multiple Margins 133

CHAPTER 5
Power and Identity 141
- Violence and Power 142
- Networks of Resistance 149
- The Albino Body as a Space of Resistance 164
- 'Être albinos' 174

Conclusion 181
Appendix: Fictional Works Featuring Albino Characters 193
Bibliography 197
Index 217

Acknowledgements

I would like to thank the many people who have contributed in so many different ways to the completion of this book. At Nottingham University, where this project was initiated, I benefited from engagement with fellow postgraduates and academics in the Department of French and Francophone Studies. Since I first began to work on this project as my Masters dissertation, developed it into a doctoral thesis and reworked it for publication, Nicki Hitchcott has generously offered much-valued intellectual guidance and professional advice. Zoë Norridge and Susan Dickinson have provided invaluable critique and encouragement, and conversations with Femi Adebajo, Nathaniel Boso and Ademola Abass provided stimulating discussions and fruitful leads. Christopher Johnson offered helpful advice on drafts of the chapters and I am indebted to Roger Little and Kathryn Batchelor, for their invaluable comments.

I am grateful to Charles Forsdick and Allyson Fiddler for their encouragement to pursue the publication of *Enduring Negativity*. I would also like to thank colleagues in the Department of European Languages and Cultures, members of the African Studies Group and colleagues in the Centre for Transcultural Writing and Research at Lancaster University who have heard and given feedback on sections of this book presented as work in progress papers. My thanks also go to colleagues in the Society for Francophone Postcolonial Studies as well as delegates at conferences in the UK, USA and South Africa who have shown such interest in this project and offered their insightful comments. I have greatly valued the opportunity to work with Patricia Lund and Julie Taylor, and I am grateful for the belief they have shown in me so early in my academic career. I would like to thank Médard Djatou, who made me so welcome in Cameroon at an important time in the development of this project. I am also indebted to the many individuals who have shared and continue to share their personal experiences of living with albinism. I would particularly like to thank Lee Edwards for his continued interest in my research.

My parents, to whom this book is dedicated, have fostered my love of literature throughout my life, showing great interest in my research and offering steadying confidence in equal measure. Finally, without the love, support and understanding of my husband Neil Cheesbrough, completing this book would have been a very lonely task. To all of you, thank you.

Introduction

Enduring Negativity sets out to draw attention to and explore the portrayal of the figure of the black African albino, and to bring about a new understanding of the potential of this figure in literary representation. The visibility of people with albinism in sub-Saharan Africa has been manipulated into a symbolic otherness by writers, film-makers and artists, aggravating the situation of individuals who are already surrounded by a web of beliefs in the form of myths and stereotypes.[1] Yet, despite the wealth of representations of albinism, very few critical studies into the portrayal of the figure of the albino have been undertaken. This study explores the different understandings of albinism communicated by three French and Francophone writers, adopting a comparative, interdisciplinary approach that not only crosses linguistic, regional and national divisions, but which also transcends disciplinary boundaries. *Enduring Negativity* draws on insights from Anglophone and Francophone literary criticism, as well as on postcolonial studies, anthropological and sociological discussions of the body, and postmodern critical thinking on the body as a discursive construct. My analysis is not only driven by an interest in the cultural specificities elucidated by each of the texts explored, but also by a wish to examine how the different literary discussions of albinism relate to one another, as well as to contemporary understandings of the condition.

The term 'albinism' refers to a group of related conditions which are the result of a genetic mutation that causes a deficiency in melanin production. Melanin is a chemically inert pigment, which is responsible for producing all shades of humankind. There are two main types of albinism, and several sub-types. Oculocutaneous albinism, which will be the focus here, results in the partial or full absence of pigment from the skin, hair and eyes. This means that people with the condition have pale skin, blonde or sandy coloured hair, light brown or blue eyes, and suffer from poor

---

[1] For a list of fictional works featuring albino characters, see Appendix.

visual acuity. The second main type of albinism, ocular albinism, entails reduced pigment in the eyes, though skin and hair can be lighter than in other family members. With the evolution of the biomedical sciences the condition has been explained in terms of genetic mutation, and health professionals are now able to protect against many of the secondary conditions associated with albinism such as skin cancers and further eye damage. Whereas in Western societies with predominantly pale skinned populations people with albinism often pass unnoticed, in sub-Saharan Africa, albinism is the most visible of disabilities. Early Western anthropologists assumed that people with albinism were found only in non-European cultures and for a time it was believed that they constituted a different race.[2] Now it is recognised that albinism is present within all ethnic groups and populations, but prevalence rates vary considerably throughout the world. As Kromberg and Jenkins note, in parts of South Africa as many as 1 in 2,000 people have albinism.[3] In specific groups such as the Tswana, who have encouraged marriage between cousins for generations, the prevalence rate is particularly high.

The language used to describe albinism and people with the condition is often problematic because of its associations. The label 'albino' is generally considered inappropriate in the West and the term 'person with albinism' is preferred because it puts the individual before the condition. However, there is no evidence to suggest that the expression 'albino' is considered derogatory in sub-Saharan Africa, where it is simply employed as a descriptive term. The expression *nègre blanc* is also used to describe the figure of the albino in French and Francophone African literature. This term is particularly interesting because of its associations. Roger Little traces three principle stages in the evolution of the term, noting that until the late eighteenth century, it was used by white explorers to refer to the black albinos they encountered in an attempt to classify them. However,

[2] Roger Little traces the first encounters with people with albinism in sub-Saharan Africa. See Roger Little, *Nègres Blancs – Représentations de l'autre autre* (Paris: L'Harmattan, 1995).
[3] J. Kromberg and T. Jenkins, 'Prevalence of Albinism in the South African Negro', *South African Medical Journal*, 61 (1982) 382–6.

in the nineteenth century, writers used *nègre blanc* not only to describe the physically white albino, but also 'morally white' blacks. According to Little, 'L'adjectif "blanc" assume quasiment de la sorte la force d'un substantif, alors que "nègre" se vide de son sens noble et [...] se cantonne à l'état où l'homme blanc l'a en réalité réduit.'[4] In the twentieth century, the term evolved once more and came to be used by black Africans to describe other black Africans who imitated their white colonisers.[5] A whole vocabulary exists for describing the figure of the albino, including a wide range of culturally specific labels. These will be discussed as they arise throughout the study, but include *dundus*, *sope* and *meffeu*.

The vocabulary used to describe the appearance of people with albinism poses its own challenges. The manifestation of albinism in non-pigmented skin makes it a condition that is loaded with symbolism and meaning in terms of racial difference. Describing people with albinism as 'black' is problematic, given their visible difference from other black Africans, just as the labelling of the albino body as 'white' brings to bear the implications of this whiteness in relation to the complex issue of race. Henry Louis Gates's position on the figurative status of race is signalled by the quotation marks within which he encloses the word. In *'Race', Writing and Difference*, Gates argues that:

> The biological misnomers and metaphors that we use when speaking of 'race' hide the dangers of this trope under the pretence that it is merely an objective term of classification [...] 'Race' is the ultimate trope of difference because it is so arbitrary in its application.[6]

Whether this difference is seen in terms of colour-based prejudice or the antithetical 'colour-blind' view that all are equal regardless of colour, the problematic assumptions about what exactly constitutes race seem

---

4   Little, *Nègres blancs*, 19.
5   Frantz Fanon uses the term 'lactification' to describe this psychological whitening in *Peau noire, masques blancs* (Paris: Editions du Seuil, 1972), 38.
6   Henry Louis Gates, *'Race', Writing and Difference* (Chicago: University of Chicago Press, 1992), 5. I acknowledge the problematic vocabulary of race, but I will not follow Gates's example of framing the term with quotation marks.

inescapable. Descriptions of people with albinism as 'disabled' or 'marginalised' are equally complex because of the dubious associations of these terms. I therefore proceed with caution in my description of the figure of the albino, fully aware of the nature of the language I use and discussing specific terms as they arise, but at the same time, with little choice other than to employ this difficult vocabulary.

Enduring Negativity focuses particularly on Patrick Grainville's *Le Tyran éternel* (1998), Didier Destremau's *Nègre blanc* (2002), and *Wirriyamu* (1976) and *Mémoire d'une peau* (1998) by Williams Sassine. These novels have been chosen because all four focus on black African protagonists with albinism and the action of each narrative takes place in twentieth-century sub-Saharan Africa. Although Destremau, Grainville and Sassine write from very different perspectives and in markedly different styles, they portray their albino characters in strikingly similar terms.

French writer Didier Destremau was born in Brest in 1937, but spent much of his childhood in Africa. He was schooled in Senegal and Tunisia before pursuing his university studies in Paris, where he obtained diplomas from the *Institut d'études politiques de Paris* and from the *Institut d'études islamiques*. In 1979, after twenty years in the military, Destremau took up a diplomatic career and was consequently posted to Kuwait, Yemen and Saudi Arabia. He wrote his first book, a study of post-Gulf War America, while posted in the United States in 1992, and it was during his time as French Ambassador to Mozambique and Swaziland that he wrote his first novel *Nègre blanc*, published in 2002. The novel opens with the birth of a child with albinism and the linear third-person narrative follows the boy's journey into adulthood against the historical backdrop of the 1960 Civil War in Mozambique. The chapters trace Samate's journey from 'Le village', through 'La savane', to his meeting with Mafavuca – a white Rhodesian soldier who adopts the young Samate on the death of his mother – and finally his experiences of 'La civilisation'. *Nègre blanc* is an uncomplicated narrative which is easily accessible to the reader. Where the novel is most effective is in underlining the great disparity that still exists in much of Africa today between life in the village and that of the city, revealing the attendant problems faced by people with albinism in each.

Patrick Grainville's *Le Tyran éternel* examines the same disparity between 'civilisation' and 'wilderness', but the novel is more complex, on the level of language as well as narrative structure. Although Grainville won the 1974 Prix Goncourt for his novel *Les Flamboyants*, his other fictional works have received relatively limited critical attention. Born in 1947 in Villers-sur-Mer in Normandy, Grainville spent his childhood in Villerville, near Deauville, before training to become a teacher. Grainville is a prolific writer and has published over twenty fictional works since the appearance of his first novel *La Toison* in 1972. He has visited Mali, Côte d'Ivoire and parts of North Africa, having read widely about these countries, and is particularly interested in politics, inter-ethnic conflicts and African myths, issues Grainville addresses in *Le Tyran éternel*, in which he re-engages with the Africa of his early novels. *Le Tyran éternel* is an ironic portrayal of Houphouët-Boigny, the first President of Côte d'Ivoire, a character represented in the novel as a leader obsessed with power, typical of the postcolonial dictators who stepped into the power vacuum left by the colonisers. The plot follows the writer Sylvanus in his search for Houphouët-Boigny's lost son, Alpha, whom he believes can challenge the political legacy of the dictatorial leader.

Grainville first came across the beliefs surrounding albinism when in Côte d'Ivoire, and in *Le Tyran éternel* he sets the taboo of the albino against the background of contemporary Africa which, he suggests, has not yet drawn a line between modernity and the beliefs of the past. The intricacy of this relationship is echoed in the complexity of Grainville's writing, which he describes in an interview with Rachel Edwards: 'Moi, j'aime le travail dans l'écriture, j'aime l'invention dans l'écriture.'[7] Indeed, it is for his use of the French language that Grainville is most appreciated, and *Le Tyran éternel* is one of the best examples of this inventiveness. As André Durand writes:

> Son ton est forcené, sa prose débridée, foisonnante, enfiévrée, excessive, orgiaque, dionysiaque, sa prolixité étourdissante. Il se plaît à l'abondance fastueuse de détails

[7] Rachel Edwards, *Myth and the Fiction of Michel Tournier and Patrick Grainville* (Lampeter: Edwin Mellen Press, 1996), 39.

colorés, aux effusions lyriques, aux métaphores monstrueuses et extravagantes, pour faire découvrir un réel luxuriant, exubérant, qu'il transcende et transfigure avec brio.⁸

Williams Sassine's writing is equally rich on the levels of language, characterisation and narrative structure. Sassine was born in Kankan, Guinea, in 1944, the son of a Lebanese Christian father and a Guinean Muslim mother. In 1961, Sassine was forced into exile in France as a consequence of Sékou Touré's regime. He studied in France for five years and from 1966 to 1988 was mathematics teacher and headmaster in several West African countries, including Côte d'Ivoire and Mauritania. During his lifetime Sassine published five novels, among them the widely acclaimed *Le Jeune Homme de sable* (1979). He returned to Guinea in 1989, where he worked as Chief Editor for the satirical paper *Le Lynx*, remaining critical of Sékou Touré and his regime until his death in 1997.

Sassine's fictional writing explores the nature of human existence, focusing on a society in crisis. His narratives pay particular attention to the human body and its degeneration, which functions as a metaphor for societal decay. The two novels examined in this study are *Wirriyamu*, published in 1976, and *Mémoire d'une peau*, which was published posthumously in 1998. These are very different novels, but there are parallels between them, notably that both protagonists have been abandoned by their birth parents and have difficult relationships with their adoptive mothers, and both characters are only recognised by those around them in terms of their albinism and its connotations.⁹

Sassine's only novel to be set during colonial rule, *Wirriyamu* offers the writer's most explicit critique of the colonial system. Focusing on the days preceding the massacre of the inhabitants of the village of Wirriyamu by Portuguese soldiers in December 1972, the narrative follows the protagonists Kabalango, a poet returning to his native village to die, and

---

8   André Durand, *Comptoir Littéraire* <http://www.comptoirlitteraire.com/files/> [Accessed 5 January 2010].
9   Pius Ngandu Nkashama, *Écrire à l'infinitif: la déraison de l'écriture dans les romans de Williams Sassine* (Paris: L'Harmattan, 2006), 141.

Introduction

the albino Condélo, who is pursued to his death.¹⁰ Sassine skilfully evokes Wirriyamu as an ordinary Portuguese colony, but traces the extraordinary events that take place over the three days preceding the massacre. The inhabitants of Wirriyamu are trapped, powerless as they are drawn inexorably towards the massacre, and the violence of the last ten years of colonial rule in Mozambique is echoed in the relentless march of the Portuguese soldiers towards the village. This is compounded by the fragmentation of the book into short sections marking the progression of time over a period of just three days.

The narrative structure of both *Wirriyamu* and *Mémoire d'une peau* is interesting. The multiple narrators of *Wirriyamu* – among them Condélo the albino, the terminally ill poet Kabalango, and Amigo, the Portuguese soldier – offer different perspectives on the action. These first- and third-person narrative voices draw the reader into an immediate engagement with the experiences of the characters. On one level, Sassine presents Condélo as a passive victim. The objectification of Condélo's body in repeated references to the ancestral practice of blood-letting and the value attached to his albino skin define him as a tragic sacrificial victim. Although Condélo is aware of the beliefs surrounding his albinism and their consequences, he is trapped in his marginality, hopelessly seeking refuge in dreams and solitude. On another level, though, Condélo is a symbolic figure, whose suffering and death on the cross render him, as Chevrier suggests, 'une figure christique'.¹¹ However, Sassine does not simply portray Condélo in figurative terms. Rather, the young boy's experiences echo those of Grainville and Destremau's protagonists, as they experience the same prejudice, exclusion and isolation, reflecting the reality of living with albinism in much of sub-Saharan Africa.

---

10   Although the Portuguese denied the existence of such a village in Mozambique, a massacre was reported widely in the press to have taken place on 16 December 1972 in Wirriyamu, spreading to Chawola and neighbouring villages. See Adrian Hastings, *Wirriyamu* (London: Search Press, 1974).
11   Jacques Chevrier, *Williams Sassine: écrivain de la marginalité* (Toronto: Editions du Gref, 1995), 214.

In contrast to *Wirriyamu*, *Mémoire d'une peau* is notable for its use of a single narrative voice, that of the murderous and sociopathic Milo Kan. Set in postcolonial Guinea, *Mémoire d'une peau* offers a critical and uncompromising view of society through the eyes of its protagonist. *Mémoire d'une peau* has been criticised for language and imagery tending towards the pornographic, and the plot, essentially a quest for love, as rather thin.[12] However, the interest of the novel is bound up elsewhere, in the complexity of Milo's characterisation and in the intricate narrative structure employed by Sassine, which reflects the progatonist's state of mind as he constantly questions his situation and attempts to come to terms with his difference. The multifarious narrative functions on three levels: the novel *Mémoire d'une peau* with Milo as the protagonist, the romantic novel Milo attempts to write, also titled *Mémoire d'une peau*, and the letters exchanged between Milo, Rama and Christian at the end of the narrative, which reflect retrospectively on the events we have witnessed as readers.

Written over twenty years apart, Sassine's two novels evoke the difficult experiences of people with albinism, conveying the sense of alienation suffered by an individual who is markedly different from those around him and the constant reinforcing of this in his daily life. Yet, at the same time, the novels express different modes of albino experience. While the protagonist of *Wirriyamu* is a passive victim of his situation, the reactive central character of *Mémoire d'une peau* is driven to anger, even madness, as a consequence of his marginalisation. In this study I draw out parallels between the two novels while acknowledging the distinct experiences of their protagonists.

Few critical studies of the fictional work of Destremau, Grainville and Sassine exist. Destremau's *Nègre blanc* has received no critical attention, and Grainville's *Le Tyran éternel* has only been explored in relation to other works of fiction.[13] Although more critical work exists on Sassine's writing, it is limited in scope. Nkashama's recent critical study of Sassine's work,

---

12   Cécile Lebon, 'Review of Williams Sassine's *Mémoire d'une peau*', *Notre Librairie* 136 (1999) 150–1 (150).
13   See Edwards (1996) and Susan Petit, '*Le Tyran Eternel* by Patrick Grainville', *French Review* 73 (1999), 163–4.

Écrire à l'infinitif: la déraison de l'écriture dans les romans de Williams Sassine is based on discussions with Sassine while both were teaching at the Université de Limoges in 1991 and relates Sassine's personal experiences as an African writer living in exile. Nkashama explores all five of Sassine's novels chronologically, from *Saint Monsieur Baly* (1973) to *Mémoire d'une peau*. His study draws out important thematic parallels, including the relationship between pedagogy and writing in *Saint Monsieur Baly* and later in *Le Jeune Homme de sable* (1997), the relevance of signs and signifiers in *Le Zéhéros n'est pas n'importe qui* (1985), the relationship between religious and mythical beliefs associated with albinism in *Wirriyamu*, and the centrality of language and narrative structure to *Mémoire d'une peau*. Importantly for this study, Nkashama's is the only book-length study of Sassine's work to explore *Mémoire d'une peau*, in which he discusses the novel comparatively in relation to *Wirriyamu*, focusing briefly on the two albino protagonists.[14]

Jacques Chevrier has published several studies of Sassine's fiction, exploring his early writing in some depth. However, his insistence on Sassine's position as *écrivain de la marginalité* – a description that succinctly expresses Sassine's personal experience of exclusion and the marginality of his protagonists – under estimates the complexity of these marginal figures in Sassine's fictional work, demanding as they do a self-reflexive questioning of postcolonial African society, and issues of power and identity. Equally, although Chevrier briefly discusses albinism in *Williams Sassine, écrivain de la marginalité*, he views the albino protagonist of *Wirriyamu* in purely symbolic terms and as a consequence overlooks the more practical issues related to albinism addressed by the author.[15]

Although Chevrier discusses *Wirriyamu* in a number of studies of Sassine's work, he has not written on *Mémoire d'une peau*. Therefore, Catherine Wendeler's article, which argues that *Mémoire d'une peau* represents a rehabilitation of the African psyche after the scars of colonisation, is a

---

14   Pius Ngandu Nkashama, *Ecrire à l'infinitif la déraison de l'écriture dans les romans de Williams Sassine* (Paris L'Harmattan, 2006), 141–50.
15   Chevrier, *Williams Sassine: écrivain de la marginalité*, 270.

welcome addition to the small corpus of critical work on Sassine's fiction.[16] Wendeler's focus on the discourse surrounding the body is particularly relevant to the present study, given the impact of bodily difference on the life of Milo, the protagonist of *Mémoire d'une peau*. The paper's only failing is that, although it sets out to examine the embodiment of wrath in Sony Labou Tansi's *La vie et demie* and Sassine's *Mémoire d'une peau*, no comparison is drawn between the two works, despite the obvious interest to be gained from doing so.

In light of the relative lack of critical attention to the work of these writers, I have found it constructive to draw on other Anglophone and Francophone African fictional writing about albinism. I refer particularly to Ben Hanson's novel *Takadini* (1997) and Namba Roy's *Black Albino* (1961) to give a comparative reading of Destremau, Grainville and Sassine's novels. *Black Albino* centres around the Maroons, a group of slaves who escaped into the mountains of Jamaica in the eighteenth century, and Ben Hanson's *Takadini* tells the story of the birth of a child with albinism into a rural village community in Zimbabwe. *Takadini* is unusual, as it was released with the support of the Zimbabwe Albino Association and provides a rather more pragmatic view of the reality of living with albinism in Africa than other fictional works. Set in the period immediately before colonisation, the novel portrays life among the Shona people, focusing on events surrounding the birth of a child with albinism. The narrative follows the life of the baby Takadini from birth through to adulthood, highlighting the beliefs that surround his existence at various stages of his life. In both *Takadini* and *Black Albino*, the appearance of a child with albinism in the community brings about a self-reflexive questioning of the traditional beliefs surrounding this figure, and echo many of the issues raised in the novels of Destremau, Grainville and Sassine.

Critical studies of the representation of albinism in works of fiction by writers other than those studied here have been invaluable. These are predominantly studies of albinism in the work of American writers such

---

16 Catherine Wendeler, 'The Embodiment of Wrath in two Postcolonial Prophecies: *La vie et demie* by Sony Labou Tansi and *Mémoire d'une peau* by Williams Sassine', *Imperium*, 2 (2001), 380–91.

as N. Scott Momaday, John Edgar Wideman and Iain Lawrence. Claudia Benthien's article, 'The Whiteness underneath the Nigger', a study of albinism and blackness in John Edgar Wideman's novel *Sent for You Yesterday*, is of specific interest because of the way in which Benthien discusses the social hierarchies and judgements associated with skin tone, highlighting the association between the whiteness of the albino body and notions of colourlessness, which I develop in this study.[17] I also draw on Bonnie TuSmith's article, 'The Inscrutable Albino in Contemporary Ethnic Literature'. Exploring the stereotype of the inscrutable albino in canonical European American and contemporary ethnic American literature, TuSmith considers the ways in which writers such as Momaday represent what she terms 'the multi-ethnic possibilities of the albino'.[18] In TuSmith's words, 'the image affords depths and nuances – moments of self-examination and transcendant insight – which the tag of white American versus black ethnic has not been able to accommodate'.[19] I use these discussions of representations of albinism to draw out and contextualise similar issues in the narratives of Destremau, Grainville and Sassine.

The notion of what TuSmith terms the 'multi-ethnic possibilities' of the figure of the albino also emerges in Ngaire Blankenberg's article 'That Rare and Random Tribe: Albino Identity in South Africa' which, she admits, is not just an essay born from academia, but born from experience.[20] The daughter of a black African albino father and a *métisse* mother, Blankenberg bases her discussion of the reality of living with albinism on her father's experiences. She explores albinism in relation to African identity, discussing the beliefs that surround people with albinism in South Africa. In particular, Blankenberg explores the deconstruction of blackness, asking

---

17 Claudia Benthien, 'The Whiteness Underneath the Nigger: Albinism and Blackness in John Edgar Wideman's *Sent for you Yesterday*', *Utah Foreign Language Review* 56 (1997), 3–13.
18 Bonnie TuSmith, 'The Inscrutable Albino in Contemporary Ethnic Literature', *Amerasia Journal*, 19.3 (1993), 85–102 (85).
19 Ibid., 99.
20 Ngaire Blankenberg, 'That Rare and Random Tribe: Albino Identity in South Africa', *Critical Arts*, 14.2 (2000), 6–48 (6).

the enduring question, 'Is the albino black?'²¹ Charles Carnegie's 'The Dundus and the Nation', which is based on the author's own experiences as a person with albinism of African ancestry in Jamaica, poses many of the same questions.²² Carnegie argues that the position of the *dundus* is one from which it is possible to question the claims to exclusiveness that the collectivities of race and nation make for themselves.²³ Carnegie has since reworked this article into the introduction to *Postnationalism Prefigured: Caribbean Borderlands*, in which he examines the 'borderlands' where nationalism, race and globalisation intersect or collide. He argues that the marginalised position of the *dundus* and the taboos surrounding this figure offer a site from which to question the inclusiveness that collectivities of race and nation claim. I will show that in their novels, Destremau, Grainville and Sassine signal a similar need to rethink the boundaries which serve to exclude people with albinism, opening up the way to a more inclusive notion of postcolonial African identity.

Although *Enduring Negativity* focuses on fictional representations of albinism, it also draws on the work of researchers in fields including genetics, the biomedical sciences, anthropology and sociology. A rich personal experience of working with people with albinism underlies the research of Patricia Lund, a South African geneticist who has published several papers on different aspects of living with albinism in South Africa and Zimbabwe. Lund draws on her experiences as a researcher in these countries, as well as her involvement in a number of recent multi-disciplinary research projects.²⁴ Significantly, Lund's work has not remained a purely scientific enquiry, but has led to initiatives which have impacted on people's lives in a positive way. Comparison of Lund's findings on the myths

---

21   Ibid., 36.
22   Charles V. Carnegie, 'The Dundus and the Nation' *Cultural Anthropology*, 11.4 (1996), 470–509.
23   Carnegie opens his paper with a definition of 'dundus' from the *Dictionary of Jamaican English* ed. by F.G. Cassidy and R.B. Le Page, 'Dundus: 1. An albino negro. 2. A freak; someone who is not up to the mark of normality'. Carnegie, 'The Dundus and the Nation', 470.
24   See for example, Patricia Lund, 'Living with Albinism: A Study of Affected Adults in Zimbabwe', *Journal of Social Biology and Human Affairs*, 63 (1998), 3–10.

surrounding albinism in Southern Africa with those discussed in the novels of Destremau, Grainville and Sassine has revealed many parallels between beliefs associated with the figure of the albino across sub-Saharan Africa. Although albinism is more visible in black populations, Blankenberg, Carnegie and Lund's papers show that people with albinism all over the world suffer discrimination as a result of the beliefs surrounding the condition. This is supported by João De Pina-Cabral's paper on the symbolic ecology of beliefs surrounding albinism in post-colonial Mozambique, Jennifer Kromberg's article which examines the response of black South African mothers to the birth of a child with albinism, Marija Ogrizek's study of albinism in Central Africa, and Pascale Jeambrun and Bernard Sergent's work on albinism among the Amerindians.[25]

Destremau, Grainville and Sassine often refer to the very practical nature of the difficulties of living with albinism and these are discussed in some depth by Abadi and Pascal in their study of the recognition and management of albinism.[26] Lund also examines the reality of living with albinism from a number of different perspectives, but with a particular emphasis on education to change the way in which people with albinism are perceived and consequently ameliorate their circumstances.[27] McBride and Leppard's study of the attitudes and beliefs of people with albinism towards sun avoidance takes a similar approach.[28] The particular value of these papers is that they draw on fieldwork conducted in Africa, and

---

25   João De Pina-Cabral, 'Albinos Don't Die: The Symbolic Ecology of Belief in Post-Colonial Mozambique' (unpublished paper, 2002). Jennifer Kromberg, 'The Response of Black Mothers to the Birth of an Albino Child' *American Journal of Diseases of Children*, 21 (1987), 455–61. Marija Ogrizek, 'Les Albinos, enfants surnaturels des sirènes: approche ethnomédicale de l'albinisme en Afrique centrale', *Bulletin Ethnomédicale* (1983), 368–92. Pascale Jeambrun and Bernard Sergent, *Les Enfants de la lune: l'albinisme chez les Amérindiens* (Paris: Editions Inserm, 1991).
26   R.V. Abadi and E. Pascal, 'The Recognition and Management of Albinism', *Opthalmic Physiol Opt*, 9 (1989), 3–15.
27   See Patricia Lund, 'Health and Education of Children with Albinism in Zimbabwe', *Health Educational Research*, 16 (2001), 1–7.
28   S. McBride and B.J. Leppard, 'Attitudes and Beliefs of an Albino Population towards Sun Avoidance: Advice and Services provided by an Outreach Albino Clinic in Tanzania. *Archives of Dermatology*, 138 (2002), 629–32.

therefore reflect the reality of living with albinism in contemporary sub-Saharan Africa. Consequently, they have provided a useful counterpoint to the fictional representations of the figure of the albino explored here.

Newspaper and magazine articles also elucidate and challenge the myths and stereotypes surrounding albinism, providing a rich resource for this study. There are too many of these articles to mention each of them here, but the titles alone make interesting reading, referring as they do to the issues faced by people with albinism in sub-Saharan Africa today: 'The Shadow People' 'What Kind of Black Are You?', 'Black Yet White: A Hated Color in Zimbabwe', 'Les Albinos victimes des préjugés', 'Living in Fear: Tanzania's Albinos'.[29] As the titles make clear, the articles discuss key issues affecting people with albinism, namely, the misunderstandings surrounding the condition, the network of traditional beliefs, stereotypes and 'modern myths' perpetuated in modern day African society, and the impact of these on the everyday lives of people with albinism.

The wealth of writing on the subject of albinism to which I have just referred demonstrates that there has been much discussion around the subject, from many different perspectives. So what does the study of fictional representations of the figure of the black African albino have to contribute? It is both astonishing and revealing that in the twenty-first century the beliefs surrounding people with albinism are still perpetuated. As Little notes, 'Les hypothèses scientifiques du dix-huitième siècle et les travaux génétiques du nôtre ont commencé à expliquer l'albinisme, mais l'imagination joue encore avec l'incertitude.'[30] Despite medical advances and a more widespread understanding of the genetic provenance of the

---

29 B. Hilton-Barber, 'The Shadow People', *Marie Claire South Africa*, December 1997, 20–4; Maryceline Masha, 'What Kind of Black are you?', *The Tanzania Guardian*, <http://www.vso.org.uk/publications/orbit/71/community.htm> [Accessed 30 June 2009]; Ronald McNeil, Jr., 'Black, Yet White: A Hated Color in Zimbabwe', *The New York Times*, 9 February 1997; J.D. Mihamlé and H. Yonkeu, 'Les Albinos victimes des préjugés', *Ana-Bia Supplement* 368 (2004) <http://www.peacelink.it/ana-bia/nr368/le04.html> and 'Living in Fear', *BBC News Online* (2009) <http://news.bbc.co.uk/1/hi/world/africa/7518049.stm>.

30 Little, *Nègres blancs*, 17.

condition, a failure to communicate or simply to acknowledge this has meant that the myths and stereotypes surrounding the condition have been perpetuated. As such, literary representation has a vital role to play in building sensitivity to the issues related to albinism amongst national and international readerships. The critical analysis of such texts elucidates underlying assumptions, opening up new discursive spaces which although lacking in immediate impact have the potential to evoke more far-reaching changes. Through the close reading and analysis of the novels of Destremau, Grainville and Sassine, *Enduring Negativity* will examine the insistence on viewing the figure of the albino in terms of constructed difference, as well as the consequences of this for people with albinism in sub-Saharan Africa. While this is essentially a literary study of the representation of albinism in the fictional work of Destremau, Grainville and Sassine, by drawing on a range of materials and perspectives I hope to give as broad a view of albinism as possible.

The postcolonial framing of this study has enabled this comparative approach. Postcolonial theorists examine the ways in which texts bear the traces of the ideology of colonialism and the legacy of the colonial era, interpreting them as either promoting or challenging orthodox views of colonialism's purposes and justifications.[31] However, as Harrison notes:

> [P]ostcolonialism is not an identifiable 'type' of theory in the same (limited) sense as deconstruction, Marxism, psychoanalysis or feminism, on all of which it sometimes draws: it does not have foundational thinkers playing a role comparable to that of Marx, or Freud; and whereas feminism, say, is first, both conceptually and historically, a political movement and a theory of gender relations in society, postcolonial studies as such seems to have emerged specifically within the English-speaking world, particularly in literature departments.[32]

As a consequence of this emergence of postcolonialism in the English-speaking world, many of the key theoretical texts drawn on here are the work of Anglophone scholars, including Edward Said and Homi Bhabha.

---

31 Nicholas Harrison, *Postcolonial Criticism* (Cambridge: Polity Press, 2003), 2.
32 Ibid., 9.

Said's evaluation of the set of beliefs which constitute Orientalism forms an important background to postcolonial studies.[33] In his re-assessment of texts from the Western canon, Said brings into question these beliefs, which he critiques as a set of false assumptions underlying Western attitudes to the East. He argues that Western writing about the Orient depicts it as a weak, feminised other, which is positioned in direct opposition to the rational, strong, masculine West, suggesting that this contrast derives from the need to create fundamental differences between East and West.

Like Said, Bhabha deals with questions and concerns raised by colonialism and considers the implications of these for culture, literature and theory. I refer to Bhabha's seminal text *The Location of Culture* throughout this study, drawing particularly on his argument for a move away from the singularities of established categories and exploration of the potential of destabilising boundaries and binary oppositions. Bhabha's discussion of the relationship between self and other is of particular relevance to my analysis of the figure of the black African albino. Bhabha suggests that it is more profitable to understand cultural differences as based on hybridities created in moments of historical transformation than to classify people on the basis of pre-existing traits ascribed to specific groups.[34] He argues for a theoretical position which moves beyond the polarities of East and West, self and other, master and slave, preferring one 'which overcomes the given grounds of opposition and opens up a space of translation: a place of hybridity'.[35] This argument is founded on the idea that resistance develops within the very interstices of a structure in which power should have erased the possibility of resistance, an idea which I apply to the discussion of power in Grainville's *Le Tyran éternel* in Chapter 5.

Enduring Negativity also draws extensively on Frantz Fanon's *Peau noire, masques blancs* because of the centrality of issues of race and identity

---

33   Edward Said, *Orientalism* (London: Penguin, 1995).
34   However, Bhabha has been criticised by some for his over-reliance on the notion of postcolonial hybridity. See Charles Forsdick and David Murphy (eds) *Francophone Postcolonial Studies: A Critical Introduction* (London: Arnold, 2003), 6.
35   Homi Bhabha, *The Location of Culture* (London: Routledge, 1994), 25.

to his work.³⁶ Fanon's groundbreaking writings on language, racism and colonialism are considered indispensable to discussions of the relationship between oppressor and oppressed, and a precursor to the work of postcolonial theorists including Said and Bhabha. Nigel Gibson acknowledges Fanon's role in the postcolonial debate, noting that '[b]y attempting to get beyond Manicheanism, Fanon was part of an emerging postcolonial debate about subjugation and subjectivity, about discourse and agency, about power and identity, about tradition and modernity, *avant la lettre*'.³⁷ Although it is important to contextualise Fanon's work in relation to its historical and geographical context, as Lewis R. Gordon et al. remark, Fanon's critical trajectory spans the political and academic disciplines of philosophy, psychiatry, social science, and literature.³⁸ Fanon's discussion of black consciousness, the body and identity, the consequences of colonial rule, and language as an index of power in *Peau noire, masques blancs* and *Les Damnés de la terre* are of particular relevance to the study of postcolonial fictional representations of black Africans with albinism.³⁹

It is important to acknowledge that a number of debates surround postcolonial theory, and more precisely Francophone postcolonial studies. Postcolonial theory has been criticised for its inclination towards abstraction, a tendency to treat colonial phenomena as more self-contained and coherent than they were (or are), and for continuing to define former colonies in relation to colonial powers.⁴⁰ David Goldberg and Ato Quayson develop this critique further, pointing out that postcolonial theory can be grouped around three interrelated clusters of ideas.⁴¹ The first is a 'desire to speak to the Western paradigm of knowledge in the voice of otherness', a move which works to destabilise the conceptual boundaries of the

36 Fanon, *Peau noire, masques blancs*.
37 Nigel Gibson, *Rethinking Fanon: The Continuing Dialogue* (New York: Humanity Books, 1999), 7.
38 Lewis R. Gordon, T. Denean Sharpley-Whiting and Renee T. White (eds), *Fanon: A Critical Reader* (London: Blackwell, 1996), 1–10.
39 Frantz Fanon, *Les Damnés de la terre* (Paris: Editions la Découverte, 1987).
40 Harrison, *Postcolonial Criticism*, 9.
41 Ato Quayson and David Theo Goldberg (eds), *Relocating Postcolonialism* (Oxford: Blackwell, 2002).

colonial project. The second is a negotiation of the affliction which means that postcolonial studies 'has to claim an object for academic study which it is obliged simultaneously to disavow'.[42] In other words, the desire to write against colonialism leaves the discipline permanently in a relationship with a past it would rather deconstruct. Finally, Goldberg and Quayson see postcolonial theory as a discipline which 'seems to locate itself everywhere and nowhere', arguing it is 'appropriatively interdisciplinary', a feature that is at once a strength and a weakness.[43]

Critics such as Anne McClintock have also signalled a distrust of the language of postcolonial theory and argue that 'historically voided categories such as "the other", "the signifier", "the signified", "the subject", "the phallus", "the post-colonial", while having academic clout and professional marketability, run the risk of telescoping crucial geographical distinctions into invisibility'.[44] With this in mind, scholars working in the field of Francophone postcolonial studies have emphasised the importance of acknowledging such distinctions, highlighting the complexities of the network of French-speaking communities, regions and countries, which come together to form a Francophone space.[45] Here I take the term 'Francophone' to refer to all cultures in which French is spoken, including France itself.

As Forsdick and Murphy acknowledge, the phrase 'Francophone Postcolonial Studies' raises many questions in itself: 'Coupling the word "Francophone" with "postcolonial" may at first seem slightly problematic, as though "Francophone Studies" was a completely separate field of research to "Postcolonial Studies."'[46] The notion of 'La Francophonie' refers to a group of French-speaking countries and regions through whose cultural, diplomatic and economic connections France maintains its opposition to what it perceives as the ever-increasing influence of English-speaking cultures. Use of the label 'Francophone' itself suggests neo-colonial segregation

---

42   Ibid., xii–xvi.
43   Idem.
44   Ann McClintock, 'The Angel of Progress: Pitfalls of the Term "Postcolonialism"', in *Colonial Discourse/Postcolonial Theory* ed. F. Barker et al. (Manchester: Manchester University Press, 1994), 252–66 (255).
45   Forsdick and Murphy, *Francophone Postcolonial Studies*, 3.
46   Ibid., 7.

Introduction

and a perpetuation of the binary divisions on which, despite the rhetoric of a 'civilising mission', colonialism depended for its expansion and consolidation.[47] Indeed, Andy Stafford considers 'Francophone Postcolonial' to be a truism, as the former already designates the latter.[48] However, the connotations of exclusion and difference which have long been associated with the term 'Francophone', with regard to the French 'norm', have been challenged in recent years and the term has come to be used more inclusively by those working within Francophone Studies.[49]

In English literature departments postcolonial studies has increasingly been challenged by new theoretical models such as globalisation theory. However, within French and Francophone Studies departments there have been attempts to draw more extensively on the concept of the postcolonial, which is recognised as a critically effective means for opening up new perspectives in the area of Francophone Studies. This has involved a degree of borrowing from and challenging of the established 'norms' of Anglophone postcolonial criticism, but scholars suggest that the emergence of a Francophone postcolonialism may be a necessary element in the interdisciplinary and interdiscursive approaches that could be viewed as the future of postcolonial research. Forsdick and Murphy, among others, argue that postcolonialism must move beyond the Anglophone stranglehold that was imposed on the field in the 1990s towards a dialogue between Francophone and Anglophone scholars of postcolonialism if it is to be truly comparative.[50]

Given the shared focus of Destremau, Grainville and Sassine on identity, race and issues of power in both colonial and postcolonial settings, a postcolonial reading of their fictional works appears appropriate. However, the study must also take account of other issues discussed by the writers that are so fundamental to the experience of people living with albinism in sub-Saharan Africa today. Therefore, *Enduring Negativity* also draws on recent developments in theories of the body, race and identity to discuss

---

47 Ibid., 3.
48 Andy Stafford, Review of H. Adlai Murdoch and Anne Donadey (eds), *Postcolonial Theory and Francophone Literary Studies* in *French Studies* 61.1 (2007), 124–5.
49 Forsdick and Murphy, *Francophone Postcolonial Studies*, 7.
50 Ibid., 13–14.

literary representations of albinism. Studies of the body and disability have often completely bypassed the albino body and even critics focusing particularly on skin have failed to discuss albinism.[51] Nevertheless, many of the issues raised in relation to other visible disabilities are very relevant to the figure of the albino.

The issue of bodily difference and identity is of particular importance to this study because in all four novels explored here, the focus is very much on the albino body, and its adequacy for the construction of identity. To discuss bodily difference, I draw particularly on disability theory, referring to recent studies which inquire into the possibilities and parameters of a critical theory of disability. These studies explore concepts of disability in relation to questions of politics and power, challenging conventional understandings which are dependent upon assumptions that characterise disability as misfortune and by implication privilege the 'normal' over the 'abnormal'. Rosemary Garland-Thomson's work on disability encompasses several of these theoretical approaches.[52] Garland-Thomson analyses the challenge posed by disability to existing social relations, exposing the means by which certain bodily configurations are deemed deviant and examining the meaning invested in these differences. In discussing the politics of appearance, Garland-Thomson examines the enforcement of universalising norms, which as I shall demonstrate here, are so damaging to the positive identification of people with albinism.

Enduring Negativity is structured thematically, with chapters devoted in turn to the albino body, myth and stereotype, inclusion and exclusion, the possibilities inherent in inhabiting the margins, and power and identity. The first chapter of the study examines the ways in which Destremau, Grainville and Sassine present the corporeal nature of albino identity. This chapter offers introductory material in the form of reflections on the albino body and consideration of the related issues of race and identity.

---

51 See for example Steven Connor, *The Book of Skin* (London: Reaktion, 2004).
52 Rosemary Garland-Thomson, *Extraordinary Bodies: Figuring Physical Disability in American Culture and Literature* (New York: Columbia University Press, 1997) and Rosemary Garland-Thomson (ed.), *Freakery: Cultural Spectacles of the Extraordinary Body* (New York: New York University Press, 1996).

Introduction

I analyse the ways in which Destremau, Grainville and Sassine acknowledge the importance of the relationship between the individual body and the body politic, identity and its embodiment, and between the subject and dominant discourse, all of which are central to postcolonial enquiry. The chapter also examines the insistently negative portrayal of the albino body in representation and the exigency of imposing meaning onto it. In so doing, it raises many key questions to be returned to later in the study, questions raised by the figure of the albino, who embodies the dilemma between the colonial need to stress difference and the desire to emphasise points of connection which is so much a part of the postcolonial world today.

The need to complete the supposedly 'inadequate' albino body and to account for what is perceived to be 'lacking' is found to be fundamental to representations of albinism. The novels of Destremau, Grainville and Sassine demonstrate that traditional beliefs surrounding people with albinism have been sustained and elaborated upon in the form of modern myths and stereotypes. Chapter 2 explores the nature of these beliefs and considers the ways in which they operate as a means of fixing individuals, groups or cultures in place, from a particular and privileged perspective. Questioning the need to explain albinism in this way, the chapter analyses the ways in which the novels challenge such categorisation of people with the condition.

Against that background, Chapter 3 examines the need to exclude people with albinism, whether physically, socially or psychologically, and the ubiquitous consequences of such exclusion. The novels raise many questions with regard to the formation of boundaries, whether these are physical or metaphorical, imagined or constructed, which this chapter examines before going on to address the consequences of imposing such limits. It addresses Destremau, Grainville and Sassine's insistence on their characters' need to 'belong', the importance of a sense of acceptance, as well as the possibility of re-inclusion. The borders and boundaries which mark the exclusion of people with albinism have long been posited as divisions between categories, but in terms of Bhabha's notion of hybridity and third space, the margin becomes a site of agency where identity can be performed and contested. The fourth chapter, then, considers the notion of the margin as a space of agency, creativity and revolution, a space that enables a subversive slippage of identity and authority. It considers the ways in which the authors celebrate the difference that marks people with albinism apart in the context of a re-claiming of the albino body.

Focusing particularly on *Mémoire d'une peau* and Sassine's portrayal of the sociopathic protagonist Milo, Chapter 5 explores the concept of marginal power in relation to issues of violence, resistance and identity. This reclaiming of power is related to the ways in which the writers posit albino identity, not simply in terms of what is lacking – which is so often the tendency in the representation of this figure – but rather in relation to the particular experience of black African people with albinism. The Conclusion then highlights the need to move beyond polarised positions on identity to account for the figure of the albino and discuss the ways in which representations of people with albinism in fictional writing about Africa bring into question the limits of postcolonial African identity.

The insistent negativity with which the figure of the albino is portrayed in these works raises the question as to whether albinism can ever be viewed in positive terms. How can the negativity associated with albinism be addressed when it is intrinsic to the very language that we use to describe this figure? In the context of postcolonial Africa, the figure of the albino raises many questions, some of which perhaps we are still not prepared to address fully. In this study, I reflect on how representations of the figure of the albino demand a questioning of the paradigms around which our (postcolonial) world is constructed. I consider the ways in which the novels address issues of race, bodily difference, identity and inclusion, while challenging the negativity which surrounds the figure of the albino. Discussing the ways in which Destremau, Grainville and Sassine posit the possibility of reinscribing people with albinism, this study considers the effect on the 'norm' or the 'centre', in relation to issues of power, when the margins are reinscribed.

CHAPTER I

The Albino Body

Despite the significant number of albino figures in literature, film and art, there has been little critical attention in these areas to the albino body, a body which, in terms of its stereotypes, is deemed racially, physically, mentally and sexually deficient and which, perhaps more than any other, has been the focus of taboo, prejudice and judgement. This lack of attention has been echoed in the failure of current discussion of the body to account for the albino body, which challenges the 'norm' and refuses categorisation. This chapter – and indeed *Enduring Negativity* as a whole – will attempt to redress the balance to some extent by exploring Destremau, Grainville and Sassine's representation of the corporeal nature of albino identity. The chapter will explore the profound consequences of asserting the negativity of the albino body for those whose normality it confirms, as well as the possibilities inherent in a body that challenges the boundary between blackness and whiteness, 'normality' and 'deviance'.

Whilst the concept of 'the body' implies a 'natural' entity, in recent years critical attention has turned to bodily subjection, appropriation and agency, which have been explored from a range of perspectives: literary, anthropological, sociological and political. There has been a marked movement away from simply writing about the body in terms of its biological state, with the focus instead on material bodies,[1] consumer bodies,[2] sexualised and social bodies, and most recently on the *cyborg* or virtual body.[3]

---

1   Bryan Turner, *The Body and Society: Explorations in Social Theory* (Oxford: Blackwell, 2008).
2   Alexandra Howson, 'The Body in Consumer Culture' in *The Body in Society: An Introduction* (Cambridge: Polity Press, 2004).
3   David Krepps, *Cyborgism, Cyborgs, Performance and Society* (London: Lulu.com, 2007).

Psychoanalytic, genetic, feminist and queer readings, among others, have demonstrated how the subject of 'the body' can serve a number of critical perspectives and the range of approaches shows the extent of the functions and roles fulfilled by the body. However, with this increased critical engagement it becomes evident that the more the body is problematised, the less certainty there can be as to what it is and what it represents. Questions concerning the body are central to postcolonial inquiry, particularly concerning the relationship between the individual body and the body politic, between identity and its embodiment, and between the subject and dominant discourse.

Albinism manifests itself in non-pigmented skin, but the relationship between the body and the skin is a complex one. There has been little agreement on where the body ends and the skin begins, or indeed whether the two can be separated.[4] Connor traces three key stages in the cultural history of the skin. For the classical and medieval worlds, the skin was everything and nothing. Connor notes that early civilisations understood the skin primarily in its role as a covering, giving the example of classical Greece which understood the skin as a layer that keeps the body inviolate. The two principal words in use in Latin to describe the skin were *cutis*, which signified the living skin, and *pellis*, which is the dead or flayed skin.[5] As the guarantee of the wholeness of the body, the skin was not itself a part of the body, but was considered to be a screen that covered the body and expressed the complexion of the soul.

Gradually the functions of the skin as integument and covering for the body began to give way to a second phase which began in the late eighteenth century, in which the skin was considered in medical terms in its narrower and more mechanical function as a membrane. This narrowing of the understanding of the skin made it possible for dermatologists to begin to consider the skin in its own terms. In the third phase, Connor remarks, with greater medical knowledge of the skin in the early twentieth century, the more general functions of the skin were not only restored, but multiplied beyond mere medical understanding, 'First a screen, then

---

4   Connor discusses this at some length in *The Book of Skin*, 9–48.
5   Ibid., 10.

The Albino Body

a membrane, and finally [...] what Michel Serres calls a *milieu*: the skin becomes a place of minglings, a mingling of places.'[6] Serres rejects the predominating notion of the skin as a surface, arguing instead that the skin is an entire environment. For Serres, the skin is the meeting of the world and body, 'through the skin, the world and the body touch, defining their common border'.[7] As Connor notes, 'skin has come to mean the body itself; it has become the definite article, the "the" of the body'.[8] On this basis, the body and skin are discussed interchangeably throughout this study, because for the black African people with albinism, the body, skin and identity are intimately bound up.

Chromatic Ambivalence

Constant references to the colour of the albino body appear throughout the novels of Destremau, Grainville and Sassine, and more broadly throughout fictional representations of albinism. Describing her new-born son as 'albâtre malin tâché de points rouges, maladif avant même de respirer' (*Nègre blanc*, 29), Destremau's Mbuya undertakes the same negative survey of the albino body as Grainville's Tetiali in his description of the albino Samate in *Le Tyran éternel*: 'Dans nos jumelles, la chevelure blanche a surgi. La peau du visage grisâtre et rose. On a su que c'était un albinos' (*Tyran*, 41). As with the albino figures in the work of Sassine and Destremau, Grainville's protagonist Alpha is defined by his (lack of) colour: 'L'Albinos, le sobriquet, le stigmate de tous les supplices. Sans prénom. Sans autre identité que sa couleur innommable' (*Tyran*, 302). Repeatedly, the suggestion is that there is no need to look beyond the skin of the albino to identify him; for it is white skin above all else that marks him apart.

6   Connor, 29.
7   Michel Serres, *Les cinq sens* (Paris: Poche, 1998), 33.
8   Connor, 29.

Although albinism is a medical condition, the manifestation of albinism in non-pigmented skin makes it a condition that is loaded with symbolism and meaning in terms of racial difference, and indeed it is often interpreted solely in these terms. The arbitrary nature of racial difference has been thoroughly explored in a corpus of critical work that, in its size alone, reveals the controversial nature of the term 'race' and its associations. As such, race will be referred to here and throughout the study primarily in terms of its relevance to albinism in sub-Saharan Africa. Cultural logic presupposes a biological foundation for race as visibly evident in physical features such as skin and hair colour, termed by Fanon, 'un schema épidermique racial'.[9] The term 'racial difference' implies that there are distinct races of people with clearly definable sets of social and physical characteristics. Yet this has come to be recognised as a fallacy, for there are no clear and fixed demarcations of people fitting coherent sets of physical traits. Instead, within any racial group there are varying shades of pigmentation, body shape, hair texture and facial structure, as well as shared characteristics across racial divides.

The modern concept of races as basic human types classified by physical characteristics – primarily skin tone – was not invented until the eighteenth century.[10] In 1735, the Swedish naturalist Carl Linnaeus included humans as a species within the primate genus and then divided that species into varieties. This early attempt to scientifically classify human types included some mythical and 'monstrous' creatures, but at the heart of the schema was the differentiation Linnaeus made between Europeans, American Indians, Asians and Africans.[11] To each he attributed inherited biological as well as learned cultural characteristics. At one end of the scale was '*homo europeanus*', light-skinned and governed by laws, at the other was '*homo africanus*', black-skinned and governed by impulse. In retrospect, the assumptions involved in these descriptions, implying as they do a descending order of authority, can clearly be recognised, with Europeans on the top and Africans at the bottom.

9   Fanon, *Peau noire, masques blancs*, 90.
10 George M. Fredrickson, *Racism: A Short History* (Princeton: Princeton University Press, 2002), 53.
11 See Adam Lively, *Masks: Blackness, Race and the Imagination* (London: Vintage, 1999), 13–54.

The most authoritative classification of the races produced by the Enlightenment was Johann Friedrich Blumenbach's *On the Natural Varieties of Mankind: De Generis Humani Varietate Nativa*, first published in 1776.[12] Blumenbach considered that all humans belonged to a single species and had a common ancestry, but also recognised that his categories were abstractions or ideal types rather than discrete units: 'Innumerable varieties of mankind run into each other by insensible degrees'.[13] His fivefold division into Caucasians, Mongolians, Ethiopians, Americans and Malays was based on what was then known about the dominant physical types on each of the continents or regions of the known world, and as Fredrickson notes, his description of each race stressed purely somatic characteristics rather than intellectual or moral traits. Blumenbach took care to refute the common claim that Africans were nearer apes than other men, but ethnocentric bias is nevertheless evident in his work. Although Blumenbach was the first to trace the white race to the Caucasus, Fredrickson suggests he did so because of the reputed beauty of its inhabitants. He then went on to hypothesise that Caucasians were the original human race from which the others had diverged or degenerated.[14]

Linnaeus, Blumenbach and other eighteenth century ethnologists had opened the way to a secular or scientific racism. In the nineteenth century further research was carried out in the West to give such racial theories legitimacy. Foreheads were analysed for shape, noses were measured and brains were weighed, all in an attempt to prove the superiority of the 'white race'. Although it became clear that there was no necessary link between physical difference and social characteristics, racial categorisation presupposed social significance in physical differences, binding the two inextricably. The demarcation of distinct, socially significant races that lies at the centre of racial categorisation fetishises the features it considers 'distinctive' and artificially injects them with social value. This does not in itself imply the division of people into inferior and superior racial groups (though that is its historical origin). It is the very practice of giving significance to physical

12 Johann Friedrich Blumenbach, *On the Natural Varieties of Mankind: De Generis Humani Varietate Nativa* (New York: Bergman, 1969).
13 Cited in George M. Fredrickson, *Racism: A Short History* (Princeton: Princeton University Press, 2002), 57.
14 Idem.

features such as skin colour, eye colour, hair or nose shape that has been racialised, revealing racial categories to be constructed, that is to say, based not on biological realities, but on arbitrary physical traits that are neither historically nor socially fixed. Blankenberg highlights the fact that race is a European invention, not an African one, and therefore its application to African identities is already an imposition. However, she notes that race and racism have been one of the most powerful forces of the century, in the guises of slavery, colonialism, apartheid and Black Consciousness, and their impact on African identities has been important.[15]

At the two extremes of colour, or race, the struggle has been to define the very nature of 'blackness' and 'whiteness', and the implications of belonging to or identifying with either group. The problem of establishing a 'norm' against which to set the figure of the albino in colonial and postcolonial black Africa is central to this study, for albinism is repeatedly set up in contrast to black and white 'norms' in the novels examined here. In a postcolonial context, such notions of 'normal' blackness are problematised because this sense of 'normality' was rendered deviant by the colonial project in its attempt to 'whiten' colonised black Africans. Notions of 'whiteness' emerge as equally problematic. For, although the history and categorisation of non-whites has frequently been subject to debate, it is only in recent years that whiteness itself has become a focus of discussion. Within white-dominated societies and among white people, whiteness remains a relatively under-discussed 'racial' identity. Terms such as 'non-white' and 'people of colour' group together racial and ethnic identities, implicitly contrasting them to the racial 'norm' that is whiteness. The manner in which black people are marked as 'black' and not just as people in Western representation has made it relatively easy to analyse their representation, whereas white people are more difficult to analyse *qua* whiteness. Thus whiteness emerges from this critical debate as multi-faceted and complex. It is problematic for it cannot simply be reduced to a dichotomous relationship with blackness, but instead emerges as polysemic. A loaded term that is tainted by notions of racial superiority, it is found to be not solely dependent upon skin colour, but to incorporate different ways of being as well as varying access to positions of privilege and power.

15 Blankenberg, 'That Rare and Random Tribe', 30.

Fredrickson traces the development of racist ideologies of the superiority of white over black, noting that before the mid-nineteenth century, Europeans did not generally regard their penetration and dominance of other parts of the globe as the result of their innate biological superiority, but saw it rather as the fruit of acquired cultural and technological advantages.[16] Fredrickson discusses James Cowles Prichard, a leading ethnologist of the early nineteenth century and a staunch proponent of monogenesis. Prichard argued against the environmental basis for the differences between races, suggesting instead that changes in the physical and mental characteristics of the races were by-products of a civilising process that Europeans had undergone, but that most dark-skinned people had not.[17] Fredrickson suggests that while such a theory does not justify slavery, it was compatible with imperial expansion based on the principle that Europeans were embarked on a 'civilising mission', which I discuss later in the study.

The enigmatic location of 'white' skin on 'black' features problematises racial categorisation according to the connotations of skin colour. Troublesome for both writer and critic, albinism raises the question as to whether or not the skin of the albino should be considered 'white'. Connor notes that whiteness has long been an ideal in Western culture, and lighter skin is still valued by women in parts of Africa and the Caribbean.[18] However, he comments that whiteness is one of the hardest skin colours to achieve, since it involves subtracting rather than applying colour.[19] Fictional writing about albinism tends to suggest that it is precisely because colour has been subtracted from albino skin that it becomes so problematic.

Destremau's *Nègre blanc* signals the possibility of misinterpreting the whiteness of albinism: 'Ne serait-ce sa chevelure rousse qu'il conserve courte et épousant fidèlement les formes de son crâne, et ses traits négroïde, à distance on pourrait se méprendre sur sa race' (241). The implications of such misrecognition are discussed later. However, it is important to note Blankenberg's warning that to interpret albino skin purely by the standards ascribed to it by European society 'would mean contextualising the figure of

---

16   Fredrickson, *Racism*, 61.
17   Ibid., 66.
18   Connor, *The Book of Skin*, 66.
19   Ibid., 161.

the albino within a racialised society, where the connotations of blackness include "savage", evil and bad; and those of whiteness include good, purity and "civilised".[20] The portrayal of characters with albinism in the fictional works studied here confirms that the whiteness of albino skin delivers none of its perceived advantages. Instead, it is consistently depicted as an affliction or a burden, and ascribed a sense of incongruity. While Sassine's protagonist Milo is described as 'ombre de Blanc, négatif de Nègre' (*Mémoire*, 124), the whiteness of Destremau's 'nègre blanc' is 'une tare' (*Nègre blanc*, 43), which gives a sense of the weight of this indelible stigma. In her discussion of whiteness, Werbner notes that in twentieth-century Europe the category 'white' has become increasingly synonymous with the European.[21] Clearly, this trend makes the notion of the 'non-white European' a problematic one. If the category 'black' is in the same way synonymous with Africans, then the notion of the 'non-black African' is equally problematic.[22]

Whiteness makes itself invisible in the West by asserting its normality, so in examining whiteness one must recognise that the constructs of 'race' and 'culture' continually 'unmark' white people whilst marking or racialising others. However, when this process of marking is considered in terms of whiteness as a stigma in black society, then colour-bound racial stereotypes and associations are challenged. In his study of Zimbabwe, Owen Sheers encapsulates the problematic 'whiteness' of people with albinism:

> On First Street department-store dummies look out onto the lunchtime workers sitting in the sun. White dummies, looking onto black people. Some of the blacks, though, are white or the whites black, depending on how you look at it. Albinos, walking down the street in wide-brimmed hats to protect their sensitive skin, blinking the fair lashes of their pink-rimmed eyes. 'Unlucky', a Rixi taxi driver tells me. 'I would not like to be one'. He laughs, 'You are black, but you are white, so you belong nowhere. Nobody likes you'.[23]

20   Blankenberg, 'That Rare and Random Tribe', 9.
21   Pnina Werbner, 'Essentialising Essentialism; Essentialising Silence: Ambivalence and Multiplicity in the Constructions of Racism and Ethnicity'. In Pnina Werbner and Tariqu Modood (eds), *Debating Cultural Hybridity: Multicultural Identities and the Politics of Antiracsim* (London: Zed Books, 1997) 226–54 (226).
22   Of course, this complexity operates on many levels, for example, in the case of white South Africans and non-black North Africans.
23   Owen Sheers, *The Dust Diaries* (London: Faber and Faber, 2004), 130.

When the whitened individual becomes the focus of prejudice within a black community, then it is whiteness that designates difference. The black African person with albinism is a 'marked white', a figure who at once replicates and defies the grouping of individuals into races based on their physical appearance.

The protagonist of Sassine's *Mémoire d'une peau* expresses the difficulty of identifying with his whiteness as he articulates the colour of his skin as an encumbrance. His body is 'un tableau signé de l'étrange, de l'inconnu' (81). The strangeness of his whiteness becomes disconcerting and problematic as the protagonist struggles to establish an identity. Blankenberg expresses this same problem of self-recognition:

> You can only imagine what happened when I looked at myself; when I glanced at me walking in shop windows, in the rear view mirrors; when I looked down, even for a moment, and saw glimpses of white and it didn't fit with who I was.[24]

The same sense of 'chromatic ambivalence',[25] to use Martin's term, is expressed by the young Condélo in Sassine's *Wirriyamu* who, holding his arm next to that of the hotel owner Robert, remarks, 'Je suis plus blanc que vous et pourtant je ne suis pas blanc' (90). That Condélo's skin suddenly becomes repulsive to the soldier reveals its colour to be troubling to the white, who sees in the albino a purer version of his own whiteness. In this moment of comparison, the albino body becomes a mockery of the white body, forcing the white to direct scrutiny at his own whiteness in a questioning of its validity as a signifier of superiority.

These references to the strange colour of albino skin highlight another tendency in the work of all three writers, allusion to the notion that this particular skin is not merely a 'casing', but rather that it is inescapable and all-defining. The novels suggest that the albino body and the interpretations placed on it become integral to the experience of people with albinism and their search for identity. It is a 'lived body' whose relationship to the realities of daily life is bound up in the systems of racism, sexism and

24   Blankenberg, 'That Rare and Random Tribe', 7.
25   Charles Martin, *The White African American Body* (New Jersey: Rutgers, 2002), 93.

ability that influence the place of the individual in the world. This form of embodiment fulfils Maurice Merleau-Ponty's phenomenological account of embodied experience in his major theoretical work, *The Phenomenology of Perception*.[26] Merleau-Ponty argues that the body is the true subject of experience, since it is through the body that we form relationships to the objects of the world. However, the 'embodied experience' of the albino is portrayed by these writers as wholly negative. For the protagonist of *Mémoire d'une peau*, the body becomes something that entraps and defines: 'Pour moi, le corps a toujours été la seule réalité, la seule évasion ou l'unique prison' (57).

Benthien explores this anthropological and ideological question of what 'colour' and 'colourlessness' mean to the identity of their bearers in her study of Wideman's novel *Sent for You Yesterday*, suggesting that the albino body shows that a concept of race based on the visibility and unambiguousness of skin tones is bound to fail from the start. In Wideman's *Sent for You Yesterday*, the character Samantha describes the protagonist Brother Tate in the following terms: 'He was white, a color she hated, yet nigger, the blackest, purest kind stamped his features.'[27] Samantha comes to understand that she must look beyond the veneer of Brother Tate's albinism to recognise the African features in his face. Significantly, she is the only character in the novel to do so.

This sense of being confined by the albino body and trapped by its implications recalls Fanon's description in *Peau noire masques blancs* of the individual who is circumscribed by the connotations of skin colour: 'le Blanc est enfermé dans sa blancheur, le Noir dans sa noirceur.'[28] Fanon refers here to the colonised body, subject to notions of the superiority of white over black deployed by France in an agenda of empire building. Nineteenth-century French leaders adopted 'civilisation' as an official doctrine and it became an integral part of how France defined her power

---

26 Maurice Merleau-Ponty, *Phenomenology of Perception*, trans. by Colin Smith (New York: Humanities Press, 1962).
27 John Edgar Wideman, *Sent for You Yesterday* (Houghton Mifflin, 1997), 37.
28 Fanon, *Peau noire, masques blancs*, 6.

in the international arena. The *mission civilisatrice* was intended to spread French culture, raising its others to the French standard and way of life in French colonies through a policy of assimilation. The aim was to attempt to transform Africans into 'French Africans'. However, this process of cultural lactification and the resulting aspiration towards physical and cultural whiteness, presupposed the superiority of French culture over all others. Therefore, in practice, the assimilation policy in the colonies meant an extension of the French language, institutions, laws and customs, and often little regard for the culture and history of the indigenous peoples.

In Sassine's fiction, cultural lactification is represented as a destructive force that distances the individual from his or her own culture, in turn forcing that individual to view it negatively. The character Américano in *Wirriyamu* is a case in point: 'Lorsqu'il était tout petit [...], il rêvait déjà d'être un Blanc. Mais il ne réussira jamais à changer la couleur de sa peau' (80). In the same novel, the poet Kabalango also refers to himself as an *assimilados*, and more specifically, as one of the first in the region:

> Ce sont les pères Jésuites qui m'ont appris à lire. [...] Mes maitres m'ont convaincu assez facilement que l'égalité se mérite par le degré de 'civilisation'. Grace à ma naissance et à mon instruction, et après m'avoir fait jurer de m'être totalement débarrassé de toutes nos coutumes, je suis devenu un 'assimilados' (80).

Kabalango recalls how he asserted his superiority over other Africans as he looked down on former friends and exploited them on his plantation. Later, when he worked as a clerk at the diamond mine, he helped the Portuguese to capture those who had run away. The *assimilados* is described as 'une espèce de batard [*sic*] ayant un peu plus de droits que les autres Noirs, mais beaucoup moins que les Blancs' (80). Américano's friends refer to him by the pejorative term *nègre calcinhas*, which Sassine translates in a footnote as 'nègre à demi civilisé' (22), highlighting the association between whiteness and the 'civilisation' to which the *assimilados* aspires. Both Américano and Kabalango fail to achieve the whiteness to which they aspire, and the middle ground that they occupy is portrayed negatively as a barren no-man's-land, rather than as a productive hybrid space.

For both coloniser and colonised, notions of the 'dirty', 'unruly', sexually deviant black – and consequently the superiority of the white – were confirmed by a policy of lactification that aimed to control and to culturally 'whiten'. Robert Young comments that the ideology and procedures of French colonialism were based on what was claimed to be 'an egalitarian Enlightenment assumption of the fundamental sameness of all human beings and the unity of the human race'.[29] However, far from the ideals of 'fundamental sameness' and 'unity', the policy of assimilation affirmed the superiority of the French in the colonies, entailing different institutions and laws for the coloniser and the colonised. Hence, the colonised would always be defined as 'French Africans' and never as 'French citizens'.

With the aim of assimilation being to culturally 'whiten' the black, the boundaries between black and white needed to be firmly imposed and degrees of 'whiteness' or 'civilisation' established. Under this system, the attempt to control the ways in which individuals perceived themselves and their relation to the world involved the control and regulation of the body and its expression. Thus, the black African body was subject to the imposition of values and prejudices, and firmly subordinated to the white body of the coloniser. The desire to maintain these boundaries is clearly illustrated in *Wirriyamu* when a soldier of the colonising forces comments: 'Mes compatriotes et moi voulons un monde clair et net. Des Noirs ou des Blancs. Mais pas de Noirs blancs ou de Blancs noirs. Nous aimons l'ordre' (158). To challenge these established boundaries would be to undermine the founding principles of the *mission civilisatrice*. Consequently, the body of the colonised became a critical site, both for maintaining colonial alterity and enacting colonial governance, and as such had to be closely controlled.

The location of whiteness on a body deemed to be 'black' threatens the all-important divide between black and white, revealing the whiteness of albinism to be disruptive and subversive. For, not only does the albino body disrupt the boundary between blackness and whiteness, but also the perceived marking by colour of the degree of civilisation of an individual. The whitened body of the albino gives the visual illusion of fulfilling the

---

29   Robert J.C. Young, *Colonial Desire. Hybridity in Theory, Culture and Race* (London: Routledge, 1995), 164.

The Albino Body

aims of the *mission civilisatrice*, as its whiteness might be perceived as the same as that of the coloniser, implying civilisation. For Martin, the figure of the albino embodies the desire of the coloniser to strip away the traditions and culture of the colonised people and to replace them with 'a duplicate "whitened citizen"'.[30] Consequently, the whiteness of the albino body is identified as a sign of civilisation or lactification, almost perversely fulfilling Fanon's declaration in *Peau noire, masques blancs* that 'pour le Noir, il n'y a qu'un destin. Et il est blanc.'[31] In these terms, the troubling whiteness of albinism unbalances the very foundations of racial identification. At once embodying and challenging the boundary between blackness and whiteness, the figure of the albino resists categorisation, challenges notions of difference and thereby undermines the constructed differences upon which the colonial system so firmly relies.

The novels of Destremau, Grainville and Sassine suggest that the whiteness of albinism is subversive in another way too. The lack of melanin in albino skin means that it displays the marks imposed upon it and references to the deliberate inscription and accidental damaging of albino skin are found throughout the novels. The albino body becomes communicative in its paleness, a chronicle of the events it has witnessed and the violence it has suffered. Martin suggests that 'White skin displays the abuse it suffers. Black skin experiences pain, but is silenced, still saddled in part with the insensitivity racial scientists attributed to black skin as a rationalisation for slavery.'[32] Benthien also refers to the insensitivity associated with black skin, noting that very early in its history, anthropology put forward the thesis that black skin was thicker than white, a property that, Benthien notes, corresponded to an entire arsenal of negative interpretations, especially a lack of feeling and numbness.[33] According to Martin and Benthien, black skin is supposed to conceal and endure its pain, whereas whiteness lays it bare. As Chapter 3 will reveal, it is in its expression of the previously hidden that the albino body emerges as one of the prime locations of resistance.

30 Martin, *The White African American Body*, 6.
31 Fanon, *Peau noire, masques blancs*, 8.
32 Martin, *The White African American Body*, 119.
33 Benthien, *Skin*, 176.

A Deficient Body

Critical work which addresses the albino body has focused simply on its lack of colour or veneer of whiteness, indicative of a more general inability to see beyond it to the person beneath. As a result, there has been a distinct failure to address the other differences or supposed deficiencies that mark the figure of the albino apart, differences that explain why the albino body is invariably depicted in representation as damaged, lacking, or flawed. As Didier Anzieu explains, 'La peau est tellement fondamentale, sa fonction va tellement de soi, que personne n'en remarque l'existence jusqu'au moment où elle est défaillante.'[34] This brings to mind Drew Leder's suggestion in his influential book *The Absent Body*, that the body is missing from our experiences of daily life.[35] Our engagement in acts of perception, movement and abstraction mean that the body is constantly disappearing from view. This disappearance is only disturbed when the body makes its presence felt when it experiences disease, pain and death. Leder describes pain as a form of dys-appearance of the body, suggesting that 'the body *appears* as thematic focus, but precisely as in a *dys* state – *dys* is from the Greek prefix signifying "bad", "hard", or "ill", and is found in English words such as "dysfunctional"'.[36] This negative presencing is characteristic of the albino body, since the physical effects of albinism, like pain, influence every aspect of the life of people with the condition.

Albino skin is portrayed in the work of Destremau, Grainville and Sassine as being at fault, failing to protect and so rendering the person with albinism vulnerable. Grainville in particular refers to the inadequacy of the skin of his protagonist Alpha, which is described as transparent, failing to protect him:

---

34 Didier Anzieu, *Une peau pour les pensées* (Paris: Apsygée, 1995), 63.
35 Drew Leder, *The Absent Body* (Chicago: University of Chicago Press, 1990), 84.
36 Idem.

The Albino Body

> Notre peau nous enveloppe de douceur et de bonté. C'est notre mère. C'est le prolongement de son ventre même. L'Albinos est nu. Il est offert. Le moindre soleil l'écorche, l'étripe, le vrille. Il est cru. Il crie. (*Tyran*, 91)

The metaphor of skin as a protective womb-like layer here conveys the vulnerability of the albino body, a reference that takes on further significance in terms of Anzieu's study of the skin-ego.[37] Anzieu's *Le Moi-peau* proposes a model for understanding the nature of the self, presenting the ego as the projection of the psyche onto the surface of the body. The skin-ego comes into being with the infant's early attempts to perpetuate or recreate the conditions of the mother's womb. Thus, any threat to the skin and to the integrity of the body takes on wider significance as a threat to the whole embodied individual.

Skin is generally supposed to protect. However, the non-pigmented skin of people with albinism is open to assault from the sun and easily becomes damaged or diseased. Consequently, people with the condition suffer from ultraviolet induced skin lesions, long term photo-damage and have a high risk of developing life-threatening skin cancer. In parts of sub-Saharan Africa, albino skin is also believed to be damaged by other factors. In his study of the beliefs surrounding people with albinism among the Ngante and Lengou people in West Cameroon, Médard Djatou refers to the care paid to the bathing of a child with the condition because of the perceived vulnerability of their skin:

> Si l'eau de bain de nourrisson non-albinos peut être tiédie au feu, celle du nourrisson albinos est plutôt tiédie en l'exposant au soleil parce que l'on pense qu'une eau chauffée au feu est malfaisante pour une peau d'albinos. Une telle peau est lavée sans frottement de peur de provoquer des égratignures qui, à la longue, se transforment en plaies pas faciles à soigner.[38]

---

37 Didier Anzieu, *Le Moi-peau* (Paris: Dunod, 1995).
38 Médard Djatou, 'L'Albinos dans les représentations et pratiques culturelles des Ngante et Lengou de l'ouest-Cameroon' (unpublished masters dissertation, Université de Yaoundé I, 2003), 79.

Rather than protecting, the skin that would generally be considered a boundary or a seam is broken down and becomes inefficient as a divide between the individual and the world.

Not only is albino skin open to damage from the sun, but it is also represented as vulnerable to the gaze of other people. In Wideman's novel *Sent for You Yesterday*, the failure of albino skin to contain or delimit is emphasised in descriptions of its 'transparency', with the skin failing to provide a division between the internal and the external. The character Samantha describes the transparency of the albino skin of Brother Tate: 'She could see through his skin. No organs inside, just a reddish kind of mist, a fog instead of a heart and liver and lungs.'[39] This transparency renders the figure of the albino subject open to the gaze of the onlooker, a vulnerability to interpretation that translates into a loss of identity. Whereas dark skin is often interpreted as impenetrable and 'concealing', light skin is portrayed as revealing and open to interpretation.

In Grainville's *Nègre blanc*, the perceived transparency of albino skin is carried still further, to the point of absence. Skin is generally considered to protect the body and its internal organs from the hostility of its environment. However, as albino skin fails to protect, to 'contain', or to carry out the functions of 'normal' skin, it is often perceived and portrayed as inexistent. In *Le Tyran éternel*, Tanella describes people with albinism as 'incomplets, inachevés, sans derme définitif' (*Tyran*, 26) and Sylvanus describes Alpha as 'le Sans peau [...] un écorché pale [...] plus nu qu'un ver' (124). The same association between albino skin and incompleteness is made elsewhere. In Hanson's *Takadini*, a character asks about a child with albinism, 'Is he not whole?', then observes, 'But no; if it were otherwise, he would not be with us' (17). The village midwife describes the infant as skinless, admitting that although she has never seen such a child, she had once heard of a baby, 'born without a skin' (14).

It becomes clear from the novels of Destremau, Grainville and Sassine, as well as the fictional work of other writers such as Wideman and Hanson, that it is in its deviance from the 'norm' that the albino body is most troubling. Its perceived inadequacies and failure to meet the accepted bodily

39   Wideman, *Sent for You Yesterday*, 134.

state distinguish it from others. Consequently it is a body defined not in terms of its own qualities and character, but by its difference. Concepts of normality and deviance contain often enigmatic and unquestioned value judgements. Whilst normality carries with it notions of convention and the sanctioning of certain states of being, deviance becomes un-natural or freakish, even exotic. Yet, deviance and normality are not independent, self-contained categories, but two sides of a contradictory and protean relationship, and so neither exists in isolation. Therefore, fictional representations of albinism invite reflection not only on the deviance of the albino body, but on the criteria that define the 'normality' of others, and this in turn communicates the social or cultural context in which these criteria operate and are given meaning.

The juxtaposition of 'normal' and 'deviant' bodies is prominent in all four novels, exposing the importance placed on normality and what is known. However, the need to see recognisable traits is constantly inhibited by the deviance of a body that fails to reflect the characteristics of those around it. This sense of disruption underpins each of the novels explored here, in which the highly visible physical differences between parents and child are emphasised and given meaning. For nearly all types of albinism, people with the condition have parents who carry the 'albinism gene', but because this is a recessive gene, it may be that neither parent has the characteristics of albinism, such as the loss of pigment.[40] The novels refer to the startling whiteness of the albino body, which is always contrasted with the blackness of the parents. In Sassine's *Mémoire d'une peau*, Milo is constantly reminded of his physical inadequacy and this is only aggravated by his mother's insistence on comparing father and son: 'Ton père, je veux dire Charles, était un homme très bien. Un bon vivant avec toujours des

---

40 Autosomal recessive is a type of inheritance of genetic traits which only becomes apparent when two copies of a gene are present. Recessive genetic disorders such as albinism occur when both parents are carriers and each contributes an allele to the embryo. If both parents are unaffected carriers of the gene, the chance of passing albinism on to their children is 25 per cent. When one of the parents has albinism, the trait will only show in the children if the other parent is also a carrier. In that case, the chance of albinism is 50 per cent.

filles. Grand, costaud, des muscles durcis... Toi, tu restais tout rabougri, tout blanc...' (*Mémoire*, 25). Milo's whiteness is equated to physical weakness whilst Charles is portrayed as strong and virile. The representation of Charles in this way fulfils Western stereotypes of blackness. In these terms, the adult Milo's extreme and perverse obsession with women might be read as a desire to reassert 'blackness', to counter the negative associations of whiteness and, in the emulation of his father, to identify more closely with him.

Similarly, the incongruous difference between the whiteness of Samate's milky white skin and the blackness of his mother Mbuya's body is emphasised as she struggles to see her likeness in her son. Mbuya expresses her horror at having given birth to a child with albinism: 'un nègre blanc, un de ces horribles individus, ni carpe ni lapin, une de ces aberrations dont la nature accouche par moments' (29). She qualifies this observation with the statement that the baby is 'une anomalie probablement nécessaire aux autres afin de goûter de tout son saoul le fait de bénéficier de la normalité...' (29). The startling whiteness of the child does indeed force the reader to reflect on Mbuya's blackness that, Destremau remarks, confirms her as a native of her country. However, in contrast to his mother's 'purity' of race, Samate is firmly positioned as an outsider, belonging neither to the blacks nor the whites. Mbuya recognises her own initial response in her husband's reaction to the child as he passes though the same process of incredulity, denial, and attempts at recognition, followed by a need to comprehend and to explain.

In the same way Makawati, the father of the baby Takadini, struggles to come to terms with his son's appearance even though the baby's condition has been explained to him: 'He had expected to see a child light in complexion, lighter than he had ever seen, but not this... *this*. He could not find words to fit his thoughts' (27). Roy's novel *Black Albino* also foregrounds the indefinable appearance of the albino baby, who is described by the midwife who brought him into the world:

> I have brought countless picnies into the world with these hands, Tomaso. I have seen those whose fathers had been *bakra* and whose mothers were of our people, but this child's face is whiter than that of a *bakra*; and its hair is like the cotton that comes from the great cotton trees on the hills. (24)

The loss of conventional points of reference means that the person with albinism cannot be recognised or classified in terms of the usual identifying features, as Grainville's Tetiali finds. When asked the age of the person he has just seen, he finds it impossible to judge, given the whiteness of hair that would normally be black, the paleness of eyes that should be dark and a skin that is damaged and flaking. 'Normal' identifying features are replaced with the distinctive traits of albinism and as a consequence the albino body is firmly positioned as other.

Disability

Dominant discourses such as those of race and physical ability are central to the othering of bodies that deviate from the norm, and writers and critics in the field of Disability Studies have pointed to the importance of understanding discourse as a means of giving meaning to bodily dysfunction or disability.[41] Bodies diverging from the constructed 'norm' serve as sites for the contentious struggle over normativity. The disability/ability system marks and devalues bodies which do not conform to cultural standards, functioning to preserve and validate privileged designations such as 'beautiful', 'healthy' and 'normal'.[42] To counter the tendency to define the disabled body in terms of its failure to meet the 'norm', New Disability Theory argues that disability is not a natural state of corporeal inadequacy, but instead that it is a cultural construct.[43]

---

41 See Adam Jaworski, 'The Normal and the Deviant Body' in *Discourse, the Body and Identity*, ed. Justine Coupland and Richard Gwyn (Basingstoke: Palgrave Macmillan, 2003), 153–64.

42 Charlotte Baker, 'Introduction', *Expressions of the Body, Representations in African Text and Image* (Oxford, Peter Lang, 2009), 1–9 (2).

43 New Disability Studies revises a previous model that viewed disability as a medical issue to be considered and managed within disciplines such as rehabilitation, psychology and other professional fields. It considers that disability is not a natural

Life in sub-Saharan Africa is difficult for people with albinism because of the vulnerability of their skin to sun damage and the sight problems associated with the condition. Although many people with albinism are registered disabled in the West since the majority are legally blind, not all people with the condition consider themselves to be disabled. However, in sub-Saharan Africa, the condition is disabling because of the hostile environment in which people with albinism live. The vulnerability of albino skin to damage by exposure to the sun is aggravated by ignorance about sun protection or a lack of access to sun creams and protective clothing. Apart from the real disability caused by albinism, the albino body is often attributed other inadequacies that are imagined or assumed, such as deafness and muteness. Moreover, albino skin is frequently perceived as a sign of physical weakness that is often further interpreted as indicative of mental inadequacy. Benedicte Ingstad and Susan Reynolds Whyte suggest that the assumption that deficit in one part of the body also spreads to others is common to all people with disabilities or bodily differences, demonstrating that people with a physical disability are sometimes equally affected by attitudinal barriers as by physical barriers.[44] The attitudes of others contribute to the problems faced by people with albinism, often constituting a more significant disability than the physical limitations caused by the condition itself.

Garland-Thomson argues that disability is not simply a physical phenomenon, but a socio-cultural one, for what is understood and accepted to be a 'disability' is always socially and culturally located.[45] Therefore, like issues of race and normality, disability cannot be understood without reference to the culture and the realm of signification in which it is experienced and lived. The albino experience portrayed in the novels of

---

    state of corporeal inferiority or inadequacy, but a culturally fabricated narrative of the body, similar to the fictions of race and gender. See Rosemary Garland-Thomson, 'Theorizing Disability' in *Relocating Postcolonialism* ed. by David Goldberg and Ato Quayson (Oxford: Blackwell, 2002), 231–69.

44 Benedicte Ingstad and Susan Reynolds Whyte (eds), *Social Contexts, Disability and Culture* (Berkeley: University of California Press, 1995), 130–8 (137).

45 Ibid., 235.

Destremau, Grainville and Sassine is firmly located in an African context, a context that aggravates an already difficult predicament. Black Africans with albinism often suffer overt discrimination that is exacerbated by a misunderstanding of the condition. Traditions that see disability as a curse or as the manifestation of sin in the family and media portrayals of people with disabilities that enforce stereotypes of dependency, incapacity and inhumanity aggravate their situation.

Destremau's description of the figure of the albino as 'hors des normes tolérées' (*Nègre blanc*, 237) articulates the bounds of acceptance and is particularly significant in terms of rural African society, where it is believed that children are still killed at birth if they are found to be disabled.[46] This threat is central to the development of the narrative of *Nègre blanc*, as it is in fear for her son's life that Mbuya leaves the village to live in isolation with Samate in the forest, a decision helped only by her husband Condé's continued indifference to the mother and her child. Mbuya recalls having heard that if people with albinism are no longer found in the village, it is because they have been eliminated, 'selon une procédure plus discrète, moins sacrificielle' (37). Mbuya remembers having seen only one other child with albinism before and recalls his sacrifice by the *feiticeiro* while she and others looked on. The narrator suggests that it is not only children with albinism who are killed, hinting that other children with disabilities are discretely 'eliminated' by the elders. While the narrator makes clear that particular beliefs are attached to people with albinism, more practical reasons are given for the intolerance of people with albinism in the village. These include the suggestion that the visual impairment caused by a lack of melanin in the eyes and vulnerability of albino skin to the sun mean that a person with albinism is unable to fulfil his or her role in the community: 'Le nègre blanc est un poids [...] Il n'est que de peu d'utilité pour les travaux des champs qui nécessitent une résistance à l'effort qu'il ne possède pas' (39). In *Takadini*, Hanson also expresses the suffering caused to the eponymous protagonist by exposure to the sun, describing how the

---

46 Charlotte Baker et al., 'The Myths Surrounding People with Albinism in Southern Africa', *Journal of African Cultural Studies* 22.2 (2010).

child screws up his eyes against the harsh glare of the sunshine and suffers from sunburn, which leaves cracks around his neck, wrists, elbows, knees and ankles. For people with albinism, prolonged exposure to the tropical sun causes discomfort, severe burning, and in the long term can lead to more significant health problems such as skin cancer.

The vulnerability of albino skin to the sun and the suffering that results from it contribute to the difficulty that people with albinism have in finding work. However, as Wan acknowledges, the main problem facing people with albinism is that many employers prefer to stress their limitations while overlooking their abilities.[47] Therefore, in much of Africa, disabled people are often excluded from education and employment, incapacitated by inadequate transportation systems and substandard living conditions. Poverty combined with a lack of healthcare and social security systems further aggravate the situation, putting the burden of care onto the family. Although Destremau's overstated descriptions of the baby Samate position him in the role of male protector, it is Mbuya who ensures the child's survival, drawing on her limited experience of village life to create a home for them. Importantly, Mbuya's thoughts are not only of feeding and sheltering herself and her child, but also of protecting Samate from the sun.

When Mbuya is killed by a cobra bite while collecting wood, Samate travels to Rhodesia with his adoptive father Mafavuca. It is with Samate's re-entry into society after years of living in exile that the boy becomes aware of his difference in the attempts of others to classify or categorise him. He is initially grouped together with others who are excluded from society: 'Sa tare de nègre-pie provoque les mêmes réactions négatives, les mêmes réticences que les lépreux' (*Nègre blanc*, 235).[48] The same tendency to group together and draw comparisons between the disabled is illustrated in Sassine's reference in *Mémoire d'une peau* to the friendship between Milo and the deaf-mute Sadou. Milo recognises that for Sadou, listening to the radio is a form of passing for normal that echoes his own tinting of hair and

---

47   Nathalie Wan, 'Orange in a World of Apples: The Voices of Albinism', *Disability and Society*, 18.3 (2003), 277–96 (286).
48   The comparison of the albino to the leper here is consistent with a common belief that albinism is contagious.

The Albino Body

skin, giving a sense of shared understanding. 'Il se baissa et alluma le petit transistor dont il ne se séparait jamais, une façon de ressembler aux autres comme moi avec mes produits de peau...' (*Mémoire*, 152). Sadou's disability is revealed only when the programmes finish and the crackling of the radio betrays his deafness. Garland-Thomson notes that the concept of disability 'unites a highly marked, heterogeneous group whose only commonality is being considered abnormal'.[49] Bodies that are disabled are perceived as being out of control, violating physical norms, disruptive in their unpredictability. The disabled body defies regulation and ordering, and challenges the concept of 'wholeness'. This explains the need to represent the disabled as one, a categorising of deviant bodies that reveals a desire to control and to categorise, recalling the grouping together of the colonised blacks by the white coloniser in an attempt to classify and thereby control.

It is the simultaneous attraction and repulsion invoked by the albino body that epitomises its troubling nature and reveals its potential to challenge categorisation at all levels. Destremau's Mbuya experiences both love for her son and revulsion at his body:

> Elle éprouve une puissante affection, une attirance sans réserve pour le fruit de sa chair, mais simultanément, une curieuse réticence, une appréhension, presque un dégoût pour son corps. (*Nègre blanc*, 104)

A similar blurring of boundaries between disgust and attraction is portrayed in Grainville's *Le Tyran éternel*:

> Mais, c'est un Albinos, un monstre. Jamais il ne retournera cette tare en sa faveur. Quoique... le tabou même, le transgresseur, le sacrilège peuvent eux-mêmes devenir sacré. Cela s'est vu. Monstre sacré! Le tour est joué. Sa différence, voilà qu'il l'érige en pouvoir. L'horreur qu'il inspire contribue à son magnétisme, à son charisme noir. (190)

In this satire of the tyrannical rule of Houphouët-Boigny in Côte d'Ivoire, Alpha's disruptive presence comes to jeopardise the tyrant's absolute control in the same way that the albino body threatens to undermine the structures

---

49   Garland-Thomson 'Theorizing Disability', 235.

upon which the colonial system functions. Houphouët-Boigny describes Yamoussoukro as 'mon corps, les lacs mon sang, la cathédrale mon cœur et mon chef' (16), revealing the intimate nature of the danger posed by the presence of the albino. The discovery that Alpha is his son, his own flesh and blood, threatens not only the power structure of Yamoussoukro, but the leader himself. For Houphouët-Boigny, Alpha represents 'une fausse note dans ce grand édifice de ma vie et de la beauté' (*Tyran*, 30) and his presence forces the leader to reflect on the validity of the moral foundations upon which he has built his tyrannical rule. Not only does Grainville portray the albino body as inadequate and repulsive in its inability to 'contain', but he also reveals it to be a challenge to established boundaries. So we are again reminded of the necessity of securing these borders, which are fundamental to the politics of identity, to concepts of self and other and consequently to definitions of normality and deviance, the same important divisions that informed France's *mission civilisatrice*.

The concept of boundaries is central to Margrit Shildrick's definition of the 'monstrous', a term she ascribes to the deviant body.[50] Shildrick argues that the presence of the monstrous reminds us of the permeability of the boundaries that guarantee the normatively embodied self. Ironically it is the very insistence on the series of binaries that define the otherness of people with albinism that draws attention to the instability of the categories that define the 'normal' individual. The albino body invites a questioning of the limits of the ordinary and the excesses of the abnormal, and reveals the tendency to stigmatise certain people as 'different' and their bodies as 'deviant'. The tendency to identify others as a threat from the 'outside' and the recurrent definition of the figure of the albino in relation to the 'normal' or the 'acceptable' is central to *Le Tyran éternel*. However, rather than setting this figure apart as wholly different, Grainville's albino character is described repeatedly in terms of a blackness and whiteness that are reversible, even interchangeable. In the words of Sylvanus, Alpha is 'ce Noir inversé, retourné. [...] Le Noir tout blanc. Le domino de Yamoussoukro!' (43). The inside/outside dichotomy is a recurrent motif in Grainville's novel.

---

50   Margrit Shildrick, *Embodying the Monster: Encounters with the Vulnerable Self* (London: Sage, 2001), 6–7.

In the conflict between the internal and the external, which are posited as transposable, the unspoken horror of the physical body is revealed. Grainville's use of terms such as 'inversé' threaten, in the metaphorical exposure of the internal, to reveal all that would ordinarily be hidden by the skin, all that is considered 'disgusting' or 'unsightly' in a breaking down of the boundaries that distinguish the internal from the external and the acceptable from the unacceptable. It is precisely this fluidity of boundaries that Shildrick attributes to the monstrous body. For Shildrick, the monstrous is never simply negative because it is never distinct, but it is always a figure of ambiguous identity.[51] The albino body is problematic precisely because the familiar is mixed with the strange and as such it is rendered simultaneously recognisable and transgressive. Thus, the figure of the albino cannot be located as wholly 'other', but functions simultaneously as a depiction of the unknown other and of the recognisable self.

The Transforming Body

As well as forming a boundary between the body and the environment, skin has taken on the role of social canvas. The albino body is particularly expressive of age, and it is constantly under threat of alteration from disease, sun damage or scarring.[52] In addition, as Sassine's *Mémoire d'une peau* suggests, some individuals modify their bodies and particularly their skin using deliberate marking and manipulation to convey personal information about themselves to others. Thus, the albino body is in a continuous process of transformation, a process that inhibits the possibility of ever fully 'knowing' it. However, not only is a constant changing of physical appearance apparent in the novels, but also an ongoing attempt to change behaviour to 'fit' or to meet the expectations of society. Sassine's protagonist

---

51   Shildrick, *Embodying the Monster*, 5.
52   Nina G. Jablonski, *Skin: A Natural History* (Berkeley: University of California Press, 2006), 65–6.

Milo manipulates the meanings attached to his body with the intention of influencing the actions of other people and their sentiments towards him, whereas in *Wirriyamu* and *Nègre Blanc*, the protagonists adapt their behaviour depending on their circumstances. Thus the albino body is portrayed as constantly active, a body in the act of becoming. This sense of the evolving body features strongly in postmodern thought, which breaks with the modern notion of a unified, stable self, instead emphasising fragmentation, fluidity, and an evolution of identity.

Such fluidity is embodied in Bakhtin's concept of the 'grotesque'.[53] The label 'grotesque' implies 'deviance' in its opposition to the 'norm' and suggests the inversion of an ordered state and a consequent undermining of power structures. In terms of the colonial project, the grotesque body threatens to undermine the notion of the compliant colonised body in favour of a disorderly and resisting one. As such, Bakhtin's concept of the disorderly body as a challenge to the existing order suggests the potential that the albino body possesses. In its disruption of the *status quo* and inversion of social hierarchies, the albino body is revealed as having the potential to disturb the social order, to undermine the colonial project and to disrupt perceptions of normality and difference.

Mikhail Bakhtin explores how, in François Rabelais's fiction, the human body is represented as a space of transformation. Ignoring the body's smooth surfaces, Rabelais focuses instead on its orifices. The grotesque body is constantly active, exceeding its margins: eating, drinking, sweating, sneezing and defecating. It continually breaks down the divide between the body and the world and represents a reassertion of the body in a challenge to the notion of the 'beautiful' classical body that was characteristic of the Renaissance period. With a skin that is constantly at risk of being broken down and eyes that are vulnerable to infection, the albino body is portrayed as damaged and leaking. The skin of Destremau's protagonist Samate is vulnerable to the sun, reddening at the slightest exposure to the sun, and he suffers from problems with his eyes, fighting conjunctivitis and other infections. The description of Condélo's reddened and damaged skin in

---

53   See Mikhail Bakhtin, *Rabelais and His World* (Bloomington: Indiana University Press, 1984), 18–58.

Sassine's *Wirriyamu* is expressed with a sense of repulsion at the albino body that pervades all four texts. The skin of the albino is 'vulnérable... à vif... toute déchirée' (*Tyran*, 116). Its failure to contain undermines the integrity of the body, threatens to reveal all that should be hidden, and functions as a reminder of human mortality.

Sassine's fiction in particular is populated by grotesque bodies, which defy classification. For Sassine, albino identity is inextricably tied to corporeality and the bodies he depicts are open, transgressive bodies that represent excess and a failure to contain. This preoccupation is particularly evident in Milo's interest in his own body and the bodies of others. Throughout *Mémoire d'une peau* he analyses other peoples' bodies and compares them to his own: 'Les corps-curiosité, les corps-attraction, les corps-charité, les corps-provocateurs, les corps-ennui' (100). Bodies are the focus of Milo's desire and his sexual perversion, and consequently function as a constant reminder of his deviance. His interest in bodies becomes obsessive and is revealed towards the end of the narrative as symptomatic of his madness. Manifesting itself in different forms that include obsessive love, extreme loneliness and the desire to kill, Milo's madness is particularly interesting in terms of the grotesque, since grotesquery is associated not only with the ironic parody typical of the carnival, but also with the external expression of a disordered inner state. In Sassine's protagonist, this manifests itself in a two-way process. Milo's deviant body is portrayed as being at the root of his madness, but in turn his madness becomes an expression of his difference. The result of a lifetime of suffering, his madness raises questions about the institutions and discourses that marginalise individuals and the assumptions upon which they are built.

Milo's madness acknowledges the profound implications of the encounter between the individual defined as other and those whose normality he confirms. The burden of definition by another is experienced by all, but is portrayed as being particularly onerous for the person with albinism. The albino skin of Grainville's Alpha fails to shield him from the piercing stares of others: 'Il sentait les sourires s'enfoncer en lui. Ça lui faisait mal. Il n'avait pas de peau, de protection' (*Tyran*, 171). Sassine's protagonist Milo is equally vulnerable and the emphasis on the gaze of the other in *Mémoire d'une peau* is evidence of the scrutiny to which Milo is continually subjected.

The definition of figure of the albino from without and the implications of this gaze underpin all four texts. Just as Milo is haunted by the constant stares that define him in terms of his external appearance, Samate must also endure the inquisitive stares of others and pretend not to hear their often – hostile remarks. Despite this critique of the gaze, interestingly the act of identifying the albino as other is also adopted by the young Milo. He describes how as a child, when he encountered other people with albinism, he would remark 'Papa, voilà un albinos' (*Mémoire*, 134). This brings to mind the child's cry in Fanon's *Peau noire, masques blancs*: 'Regarde le nègre! J'ai peur!'[54] Like Fanon's child, Milo attempts to confirm his normality by labelling the other. Yet the similarity is superficial. For whereas Fanon refers to the weight of definition from without that implies responsibility for his body, his race and his ancestry, Milo's is a denial of the likeness he sees in other albinos and a refusal of association with them.

Freakery

In the process of identification from without, the albino body becomes a spectacle, defined by its difference, to be stared at or gazed upon. The desire to look at the deviant body is a paradoxical human need and one that was fulfilled in the exhibition of anomalous bodies that constituted the Freak Show. In the Freak Shows of the nineteenth and early twentieth centuries, people with albinism were put on show to the public alongside other 'freaks of nature', including conjoined twins, dwarfs and giants. The freaks displayed appealed to people's curiosity for the unknown and satisfied the simultaneous attraction and repulsion of the diseased and deformed, allowing people to confront extreme forms of otherness. Although at once fascinating, disgusting, attractive and repulsive to the onlooker, so troubling are these bodies that they can only be accepted if placed at a safe distance.

54 Fanon, *Peau noire, masques blancs*, 90.

The Albino Body

In her study of freakery, Garland-Thomson notes that the extraordinary body is fundamental to the narratives by which we make sense of ourselves and our world.[55] She argues that much can be learned from the curious mixture of fascination and repulsion with which people defined as freaks are greeted by scholars and the general public. Hall also asserts that identities are constructed through, not outside, difference.[56] This entails the recognition that the positive meaning of any term can only be constructed in relation to the other, or the 'negative', and explains the fascination with the deviant bodies on display in the Freak Show. In permitting an encounter with the other, whilst maintaining the extreme difference of the so-called 'deviant' body, the Freak Show preserves the distance necessary for the anomalous body not to pose a threat to the 'normality' of the onlooker.

Although the Freak Show vanished after the Second World War, images of freaks, whether grotesque, horrific or amusing, reappeared in literature, the media and the arts, as well as in fairs and circuses. The same terror and fascination inspired by the original Freak Shows continues today in the attention of the media to the deviant body. In the United Kingdom, the 2004 documentary 'Mutants' featured people with albinism in its third episode and the 2005 series 'Body Shock' portrayed people's experiences of living with albinism, which it described as one of the 'extremes' of the human body. Most recently, in 2009 'Britain's Whitest Family' focused on the lives of three people with albinism in contemporary Britain and in June 2010, the documentary 'Albino United' told the story of a Tanzanian football team made up of young men with albinism who set out to prove to the country that they are able to play a positive role in society.[57] This contemporary resurgence of the Freak Show in the attention of the media to the anomalous body proves its ability to address such contentious designations as 'abnormal' and 'deviant', and the role of such terms in confirming the normality of others.

---

55 Garland-Thomson, *Freakery*, 1.
56 Hall, *Questions of Cultural Identity*, 5.
57 'Mutants' (Channel 4, June, 2004); 'Body Shock' (Channel 4, February, 2005); 'Britain's Whitest Family' (Channel 4, September 2009); 'Albino United (Channel 4, June 2010).

Despite the incessant gaze upon the albino body, there is repeated reference in the texts explored here to a failure to see beyond the surface of albino skin, a failure to identify (and identify with) the albino individual. The protagonist of *Nègre blanc* is frustrated at the inability of others to acknowledge him, expressing the alienation, the social anxiety and the loneliness that characterise what it can mean to be a person with albinism: 'Sa sensibilité est blessée par l'inaptitude des premiers hommes rencontrés à le regarder en face et à ne considérer en lui qu'un être affligé d'une tare disgracieuse, qui l'exclut du genre humain' (*Nègre blanc*, 236). This inability to see beyond albinism is commonplace and an unwillingness to associate with people with the condition is found throughout fictional representations of albinism. In Hanson's *Takadini*, the *mbira* player Kutukwa promises the boy's adoptive father that he will teach Takadini to play the instrument, but it is not until some time later that Kutukwa eventually finds the courage to approach the child. He tells Takadini's mother, 'I am a little bit afraid of your boy, Ambuya, so I did not come. He scares me, as if he is not from this world. He is a stranger among us, I tell you, a stranger' (137).

An inability to see beyond the external manifestation of albinism is also clear from the language used to describe each of the protagonists. Alpha and Condélo are simply referred to as 'l'Albinos' (*Tyran* 91, *Wirriyamu* 27), Hanson's Takadini is 'sope' (*Takadini* 12), Roy's Tomaso is labelled 'dundoes' (*Black Albino* 25), and in *Nègre blanc*, Destremau's Samate is alternately labelled 'l'albinos' (79) and 'le nègre blanc' (29). The only protagonist to challenge his labelling as 'albino' is Milo in *Mémoire d'une peau*. He tells his wife that she should identify herself as the wife of Milo Kan, the albino (*Mémoire*, 45). In so doing, Milo acknowledges the refusal of others to look beyond the exterior and to identify people with albinism as individuals. The label of 'albino' is sufficient, conveying in one word the extreme difference that marks him apart. Leonard Cassuto explores this process of labelling in his analysis of the racial grotesque, which centres on what he terms 'racial objectification'. 'the attempt to turn a person into a thing on the basis of race'.[58] In colonial society, the tendency was to objectify the

---

58 Leonard Cassuto, *The Inhuman Race: The Racial Grotesque in American Literature and Culture* (New York: Columbia University Press, 1997), xiii.

colonised; hence the 'racial grotesque' was created from the fusion between object and human. The same process of objectification reinforces the distance necessary for people with albinism to be identified without posing a threat to those who consistently define them as other.

Not only are people with albinism subject to the stares of others, but also to more overt manifestations of the very prejudices encouraged and satisfied by the Freak Show. Bullying and abuse underlie all four texts, but are most overt in *Mémoire d'une peau*. Milo's childhood in particular is overshadowed by both positive and negative discrimination as people react to him by either rejecting him, by over-acceptance, or with obvious embarrassment: 'Je revoyais en un éclair mon enfance. Les camarades qui m'insultaient, les maîtres qui ne m'envoyaient jamais au tableau, les filles qui avaient peur de m'approcher' (*Mémoire*, 25). The young Milo is the victim of physical and psychological abuse that continues in many guises throughout his adult life, so that events such as a meal at the Andréas's house become '[un] jeu de ping-pong hebdomadaire dans lequel je tenais le rôle de balle' (*Mémoire*, 11). Milo's life is defined by the back and forth negotiation of identity as he repeatedly finds himself literally and metaphorically 'caught in the middle'. Despite attempts to deal with the constant stream of remarks from others, Milo's ultimate avoidance of situations in which this might occur reveals the potential threat they pose.

The consequence of the bullying and abuse suffered by the protagonists is a constant reinforcing of difference, which results in alienation and ultimately withdrawal. Avoidance of the gaze of the other is evident in all four narratives as Condélo, Samate and Alpha take to the forest or savannah, whilst Milo deliberately avoids situations in which he will be the centre of attention. Milo repeatedly expresses his desire to escape the gaze of others, something that is possible only when attention is drawn away from him. He recalls how under the old order, he always felt happy when mass arrests were taking place and others were for once the centre of attention: 'C'était les autres qu'on montrait du doigt. Moi, on m'avait assez vu' (134). Fanon articulates the shared desire of all those who are marginalised to be determined as simply 'un homme, rien qu'un homme,'[59] free of the labels

---

59 Fanon, *Peau noire, masques blancs*, 64.

and associations that mark individuals apart. It is precisely the possibility of being 'other than albino' that haunts Milo, inspiring his fantasies and, in his failure to realise them, his vengeance.

While a propensity for hyperbole in writing about albinism reveals how writers struggle with the inadequacy of language for the expression of albinism and the depiction of people with the condition, Sassine is conscious of the distorting power of language, and plays with this in his writing. In the opening pages of *Mémoire d'une peau* he highlights the inadequacy of language in references to Milo's inability to express himself:

> C'était un lundi comme tous les lundis que Dieu me donne. J'ai essayé de noter mais les mots, avant d'arriver au bout des doigts, disparaissaient bousculés par d'autres mots, qui tombaient à leur tour, n'exprimant rien de bien nouveau ni de bien solide. (*Mémoire*, 13)

The opening sentence is repeated throughout the narrative, suggesting that this struggle is an ongoing one. Milo's comment that the albino is 'comme une luciole dans la nuit' (81) is typical of the hyperbolic language, replete with similes and metaphors, that is used by the writers and which bears witness to the difficulty of defining the figure of the albino. The image of the firefly here gives some sense of the ephemeral nature of this figure, which is also emphasised by Grainville in his description of Alpha as 'ce fuyard unique, cet exilé mystérieux' (*Tyran*, 28) and 'le Blême, le Tout Autre, ce fils affabulé, ce rebut de chimère' (248). Such attempts to define the albino fail to do more than further confirm his ambiguous nature and reveal the most fundamental problem implicit in writing the taboo or marginal identity to be the impossibility of 'knowing' the other. Milo's subversive language, which includes debased and obscure dialogue and even silence, is also evidence of Sassine's manipulation of language, serving to augment the effects of Milo's subversive corporeality.

This struggle to represent the figure of the albino is also evident in the misrepresentation of albinism that occurs as a result of the refusal or failure of writers of fiction to address certain issues. The most significant of these is the poor eyesight of people with the condition and one of the few references is found in a description of Condélo's 'petits yeux myopes' (50) in Sassine's *Wirriyamu*. The very brevity of the mention implies a lack of interest and dramatic potential in the fact of his visual impairment. Characteristic of much writing about disability, the sexuality of a body deemed 'disabled' is also ignored, or in Milo's case is portrayed at the other extreme as a perverse sexuality that is equally deviant. Sexuality is very much associated with youth and physical attractiveness, and when it is not it is often considered less acceptable. Repeated instances of events being glossed over are found. Aspects of albinism that are not 'appropriate' to the writer's particular portrayal of albinism are sidestepped and, of course, there is the natural tendency of representation towards stereotyping and the expression of prejudice, which will be discussed in the following chapter. Even Destremau's attempt to explain his reasons for writing about albinism appears sentimentalising:

> Ce livre n'est ni une ode à l'albinisme, ni un traité sur cette maladie congénitale frappant de nombreux Africains. Mais, pour avoir trop souvent rencontré de ces pauvres enfants clignant des yeux sous le soleil ou de ces courageux adultes privés de pigment dermique et souffrant gravement des iris, j'ai voulu, à ma manière, réhabiliter l'humanité de 'ceux qui voient la nuit' comme le monde les qualifiait il n'y a pas si longtemps encore... (*Nègre blanc*, 3)

Although the tendency of representation to distort and misinterpret, to amplify and to misrepresent is evident in these narratives, Harrison reminds us that whereas a historian is obliged both to be accurate and to make his or her perspective clear, the obligations of the author of fiction towards the reality that he or she depicts, and towards his or her readers are less clear-cut.[60] Edward Jayne also asserts that misrepresentation is a natural constituent of fiction, for unless the truth is distorted or reorganised, fiction cannot, by definition, be fiction.[61] The misrepresentation of albinism in these novels may simply be the consequence of such tendencies, since the albino body, in its perceived 'lack', invites interpretation and inspires elaboration. However, it is significant that such negativity is persistent across all fictional writing about albinism, as well as in other forms of

---

60 Harrison, *Postcolonial Criticism*, 3.
61 Edward Jayne, *Negative Poetics* (Iowa City: University of Iowa Press, 1992), <http://www.uiowa.edu/uiowapress/jaynegpoe.htm> [Accessed 21 June 2009].

representation. When knowledge is absent, fiction becomes a substitution for the unknown. Even critics and writers who on the surface appear to have researched the condition are frequently revealed as being misinformed or as tending to generalise. For example, Martin's sweeping statement that 'the skin conditions of albinism and vitiligo cause little or no physical debilitation' is typical of misunderstandings about albinism.[62] It is possible that the propensity towards misrepresentation and a failure to portray a positive image of albinism are due to the fact that without any fiction written by people with the condition, there is no alternative model of representation. However, the legacy of colonialism and the wealth of meanings attached to albinism mean that to consider the condition from any culturally specific position would be to ignore the wider significance of the negativity with which albinism is represented.

---

62   Martin, *The White African American Body*, 187.

CHAPTER 2

Myth and Stereotype

Given the vulnerability of the albino body to interpretation, the frequency of references in the work of Destremau, Grainville and Sassine to the stereotypes and myths that surround the figure of the albino is unsurprising. Overtly stereotypical representations of albinism suggest that the need to account for what is perceived to be 'lacking' is a fundamental concern of fictional writing about this figure. The works of these three authors demonstrate that albino identity is created, imposed and contested, and in each case problematised by the web of myths, beliefs and stereotypes that have long surrounded albinism. Traditional beliefs, by which I mean beliefs which preceded and continued to run parallel to those introduced by the coloniser, have been sustained and elaborated upon in the form of modern myths and stereotypes, devices of 'marking apart' that stigmatise people with the condition. The consequences are profound. As Robert Murphy notes, 'the greatest impediment to a person's taking full part in his society is not his flaws, but rather the tissue of myths, fears and misunderstandings that society attaches to them'.[1] This chapter explores the fabrication of the stigma of albinism, the process and consequences of categorisation through stereotyping, and the difficulties that ensue for the stereotyped or stigmatised individual. It will be argued that the portrayal of the figure of the albino is bound up in these stereotypes and that the (im)possibility of discrediting or declining such fixed forms of representation problematises the constitution of albino identity.

---

1   Robert Murphy, 'Encounters: the Body Silent in America', in *Disability and Culture* ed. by B. Ingstad & S.R. Whyte (New York: Henry Holt, 1995), 140–58 (140).

The Stereotypes of Albinism

Destremau, Grainville and Sassine's novels demonstrate that stereotyping operates on different levels. The nature of stereotypes has received considerable critical attention and a clear consensus emerges concerning the damaging effects of this all-determining categorisation of individuals, groups and cultures. Of the critics who have addressed the process of stereotyping, albeit from different standpoints, Michael Pickering, Mireille Rosello and Charles Stangor concur that stereotypes are simplistic, rigid and based on discriminatory values, and that the act of stereotyping is an aggressive act of definition.² In the guise of such culturally fabricated myths of the body as race, disability and gender, stereotypes forge and manipulate evidence to promote prejudice, even when that is not the intention. The assertion and repetition of certain characteristics of an individual or group often means that they come to be accepted as unquestioned facts. While stereotypes occur in all types of discourse and draw upon various ideological assumptions, they operate as a means of fixing individuals, groups or cultures in place from a particular and privileged perspective. In so doing, they function as what Bhabha terms 'co-ordinates of knowledge', that is to say, 'modes of differentiation, defence, fixation and hierarchisation'.³

Creating an illusion of order, stereotypes lock groups and individuals into place in terms of an apparently secure framework of relations, creating and reinforcing prejudice, serving only to protect those who promote them. Rosello clarifies this, commenting that '[i]n the presence of a stereotype, you are asked implicitly or explicitly to approve, to agree, to nod, and to feel understood and properly positioned as a legitimate member

---

2   Michael Pickering, *Stereotyping: The Politics of Representation* (Basingstoke: Palgrave, 2001); Mireille Rosello, *Declining the Stereotype: Ethnicity and Representation in French Cultures* (Dartmouth: University of New England Press, 1997); Charles Stangor, *Stereotypes and Prejudice: Essential Readings* (London: Psychology Press, 2002).
3   Homi Bhabha 'The Other Question: Stereotype, Discrimination and the Discourse of Colonialism' in *The Location of Culture*, 66–84 (72).

Myth and Stereotype

of a group whose identity is well defined and legitimately celebrated'.[4] It is almost impossible to remain outside of the stereotype and this contributes to its very complexity.

There has, however, been some argument in favour of stereotypes.[5] One might argue that stereotypes are grounded in truth and therefore facilitate the transmission of ideas, images and concepts. More controversially, Jack Nachbar and Kevin Lause describe the process of stereotyping as 'a natural method of classification, an attempt to 'know' the other by means of generalisation'.[6] They contend that, in the absence of sufficient information about a group or individual, the missing information may be substituted with stereotypical discourse. Stereotypes can also be seen to function as a series of alternative selves, which offer possibilities for the marginalised individual. In sociological terms, the notion of 'possible selves' represents an individual's ideas of what they might become, would like to become, or what they fear becoming. However, I use the term here to refer to the possibility of alternative identities – multiple interpretations of the identity of an individual who is perceived in different ways by different people. When one aspect of an individual's identity becomes problematic, the possibility of associating with a more favourable stereotype becomes a form of agency. Equally, a stereotype perceived as negative by one group or culture can be viewed more positively by another, so the switching of allegiance from one group to another constitutes a manipulation of stereotypes to the benefit of that individual. Thus, the stereotype becomes an apparatus that enables an individual to shape his or her identity by aligning him or herself with certain groups when discredited by others. This layering of identities is illustrated most clearly by the *métis* individual who might associate with different racial groups depending upon the situation, playing to the criteria of acceptability at any one time.

---

4   Rosello, *Declining the Stereotype*, 11.
5   Ibid., 23.
6   Jack Nachbar and Kevin Lause, *Popular Culture: An Introductory Text* (Ohio: Bowling Green University Popular Press, 1992), 21–5.

With regard to the novels of Destremau, Grainville and Sassine, the interest is not simply in the positive or negative connotations of stereotypes. It is the process of subjectification that results from stereotypical discourse that is of interest, because whether negative or positive, stereotypes emerge as expressions of beliefs and values. It is in the creation of a dichotomy between self and other – the identification of the other and in turn the assertion or confirmation of the security of the self – that the logic of exclusion and containment behind stereotypes becomes evident. In Sassine's *Wirriyamu*, Condélo understands the stereotyping of the other to be necessary in the construction of his difference, because in turn it valorises the normality of others:

> Je savais que tu ne m'abandonnerais pas. Parce que, toi, tu le sais: je ne suis ni fou ni mauvais. Les hommes, ils sont tous comme ça: ils ont besoin d'avoir chacun leur fou. Parce qu'à côté d'un fou, ils se gonflent et remercient le ciel… (30)

Pickering argues that stereotyping constructs difference as deviant for the sake of normative gain, exaggerating and homogenising those traits held to be characteristic of particular categories.[7] Stereotypes serve as blanket generalisations for all individuals assigned to such categories and the images and notions associated with them are then consensually shared in the interests of the group among whom they are most widely used. For example, stereotypes of Africans have long been constructed by Europeans, valorising whiteness while marginalising blackness with the consequence of producing and affirming their subordinate position. In the same way, Africans have long held stereotypes of Europeans, although as Mia Bay observes, these serve an altogether different purpose.[8]

The novels demonstrate that the ordering that stereotyping produces is always at a cost to those who are stereotyped, so is damaging to an individual's social and personal identity. The fixing of individuals into a marginal position or the imposition of a subordinate status means that they are judged accordingly, regardless of the inaccuracies of that stereotype.

---

7   Pickering, *Stereotypes*, 3.
8   Mia Bay, *The White Image in the Black Mind* (Oxford: Oxford University Press, 2000), 75–117.

Myth and Stereotype

The stereotypical insistence on the homogeneity of groups that is fundamental to the marking of deviance results in a loss of individuality for the stereotyped individual, a notion that is expressed repeatedly in fictional writing about albinism. As Destremau's Mbuya reflects on the little she knows about people with the condition, she attributes one trait to all people with the condition:

> On disait d'eux qu'ils portaient le mauvais œil, justement parce qu'ils pouvaient voir la nuit, non seulement les choses mais surtout les forfaits qu'accomplissaient les êtres humains à l'abri de l'obscurité, de même que ce qu'ils concoctaient au tréfonds de leurs âmes. (*Nègre blanc*, 30)

In the same way, although discussion in Grainville's *Le Tyran éternel* at the time centres on one particular individual, Dje Dje makes the generalising remark: 'les albinos n'ont pas bonne presse. Ils portent poisse' (88). It is precisely because stereotypes portray particular groups or categories as homogeneous that they are usually considered inaccurate. Bhabha argues that in denying the colonial subject 'negative difference', he is also denied individuality, for the uniqueness of the stereotyped subject is refused, 'a form of negation which gives access to the recognition of difference'.[9] In the same way, the failure to acknowledge difference in the rush to categorise is illustrated by a repeated definition of people with albinism as no more than albino; a denial of originality and selfhood. However, Sassine's protagonist Milo manipulates this homogeneity into a characteristically cynical articulation of solidarity, asserting: '*Nous* préférons la nuit à la lumière...' (*Mémoire*, 134).

For Bhabha, it is the very act of 'fixing' the other in terms of his or her difference that functions as a denial of 'original' identity in favour of the racial and cultural hierarchisation upon which colonial power is founded. Bhabha argues that the colonial system of defining the other involved the grouping together of the colonised, construing them as 'a population of degenerate types on the basis of racial origin in order to justify conquest and to establish systems of administration and instruction'.[10] In terms of

---

9 Bhabha, 'The Other Question', 75.
10 Ibid., 70.

the individual with albinism though, the denial of identity is not only that of the colonised denied individuality by the coloniser, but also of the black African denied blackness and the whitened black denied access to the white world. Excluded from positions of blackness and whiteness, the albino is, in Destremau's words, 'un paria parmi les Noirs, et un simulacre, une pâle copie pour les Blancs' (*Nègre blanc*, 256). Destremau suggests that the only way in which the albino can be known is when defined in terms of categories that are already understood, in this case, blackness and whiteness.

Bhabha describes the stereotype as 'the major discursive strategy of "fixity", which defines the other in terms which are unchanging, knowable and predictable'.[11] In a point that is particularly pertinent to albinism, he argues that fixity is a mode of representation that connotes rigidity and predictability, exposing the fear of disorder and degeneracy that would occur in its absence.[12] As we have previously acknowledged, the albino body threatens to break down boundaries and to expose the fallacies of race, disability and in turn, notions of normality. Stereotypes are constructions that result in the production of a shadow of the other, which is adequate only to ensure that differences between the 'normal' and the 'deviant' are recognised and maintained. For Bhabha, the stereotype is not a simplification because it is a false representation of a given reality, but because it is an arrested, fixated form of representation.[13] This concept of 'fixing' illustrates most succinctly that a stereotype can best be understood as a frozen, immutable image. However, despite its unchanging nature, the stereotype functions as a form of knowledge that 'vacillates between what is always in place, already known, and something to be repeated'.[14] It is the very repetition of the stereotype that undermines its fixity, for the stereotype is not the same each time it is repeated. Instead, its implications vary according to the historical moment, as do the circumstances surrounding its repetition and the individual expressing that stereotype. These variations in the interpretation of the fixed stereotype constitute its ambivalence.

11   Ibid., 66.
12   Idem.
13   Ibid., 75.
14   Idem.

Sassine's *Mémoire d'une peau* demonstrates that the historical contingency of stereotypes means that a designation which is positive at one point in time can be seen as negative at another as values change. Although the novel is set in postcolonial Africa, it refers back to a pre-colonial time when superstition is posited as being at the root of the beliefs surrounding albinism. In this novel, the confrontation between the 'traditional' beliefs surrounding albinism and Milo's modern-day life in which they are still enforced results in a conflict of identity for the protagonist. Equally, the cultural relativity of stereotypes is repeatedly signalled by references to the acceptability or otherwise of certain attributes assigned to people with albinism. This is particularly evident in secondary material that refers to the veneration of people with the condition for specific reasons in some African societies and the exclusion of them on the same basis in others, a phenomenon which I will discuss later in this chapter. As previously acknowledged, the very contingency of stereotypes offers the potential for the stereotyped individual to manipulate the process of categorisation that defines them. Such contingency makes it possible for individuals to align themselves more closely with groups that view the stereotypes that define them in a more positive way.

The different values attached to the stereotypes of albinism make them difficult to discuss in generalising terms. However, it is the fact that the same characteristics are recurrently seized upon that is of interest, whether they are given positive or negative value, since these are the *differentia* that are perceived to set people with albinism apart. The most common stereotypes surrounding albinism are based upon the distinctive appearance of people with the condition. The striking appearance of people with albinism has for centuries been a source of fascination and today a plethora of misconceptions about the condition persists. The qualities of albinism are often given to characters in literary and visual representation to identify them as deviant or strange. Bizarre characters – usually villains – labelled 'albinos', with white skin and hair, and blood-red eyes plague the entertainment industry. Albino figures populate science fiction films and comics, and pale-skinned, white-haired characters are often found inhabiting the realm of Faerie, usually taking the form of nymphs or winter queens. The features considered to be characteristic of albinism are exaggerated for dramatic effect and in many cases albino characters are endowed with supernatural powers and other qualities that serve to emphasise their abnormality. This is a trend that contributes to the difficulties faced by people with albinism, for it compounds the tendency of others to regard them as freaks of nature, or objects of curiosity.

The most common stereotype that people with albinism have red eyes does not appear in the work of Destremau, Grainville or Sassine.[15] However, as noted in the previous chapter, frequent references to the startling whiteness of albino skin can be found in each of the narratives as well as other fictional accounts of albinism. While the skin of Destremau's Samate is described as 'la peau blanc laiteux' (*Nègre blanc*, 30), Alpha's skin is 'blanc comme un asticot' (*Tyran*, 233), Milo refers to his own 'sale tête blanche' (*Mémoire*, 8), and the protagonist of Yves Pinguilly's short story, *Manèges dans le désert*, is described as 'plus blanc que blanc'.[16] The description of Condélo's skin as 'si blanc', that apparently marks him as 'un albinos cent pour cent' (*Wirriyamu*, 50) is one of only two allusions in the texts to the varying levels of pigmentation of albino skin that determine the type and degree of albinism. The second of these is found in Destremau's *Nègre blanc* where Samate is described as a 'nègre-pie' (235), but this is the sole mention of piebaldism and as such appears to be a mis-reading of his albinism.[17] Elsewhere in the work of Destremau, Grainville and Sassine, as well as in other fictional writing in which people with albinism are portrayed, the assumption is that the whiteness of albinism is uniform and unchanging.

---

15   With different types of albinism the amount of pigment in the eyes varies. Most people with albinism have greyish, light blue or brown eyes.
16   Yves Piguilly, *Manèges dans le désert* (Paris: Editions Nathan/HER, 2001), 66.
17   Piebaldism is a rare disorder of melanocyte development. Although piebaldism can be classed as partial albinism, eye pigmentation is normal so the vision problems associated with albinism are not present.

Alternative Explanations

Destremau, Grainville and Sassine do not discuss the genetic ætiology of albinism, echoing (and perhaps contributing to) the fact that despite the wealth of research and documentation on the genetic nature of albinism, a failure to communicate this has resulted in the continued misunderstanding that surrounds the medical condition. In their population study of oculocutaneous albinism in South Africa, Lund et al. found widespread ignorance of the condition. Seventy-four per cent of the four hundred respondents questioned in their study indicated that they did not know what caused albinism.[18] The consequence of this lack of knowledge is a misinterpretation of the condition. Stine Hellum-Braathen and Benedict Ingstad's study of albinism in Malawi discusses some of the most common attitudes and beliefs related to albinism, which stem from such ignorance of the genetic cause of the condition. They record how one mother, when asked why she thought she had a child with albinism, responded: 'Maybe it's an illness in me, that's why I gave birth to him.'[19] Lund also highlights the lack of understanding of the condition among health professionals, which contributes to such misconceptions:

> I asked a local health professional about the disease [...]. He told me that it is a skin disease which can cause illness in new-born children if the mother has the disease when she is giving birth.[20]

One of the most common misconceptions about albinism is that it is contagious. The association of albinism with leprosy in Destremau's *Nègre blanc* reflects this notion: 'Samate [...] inspire malaise et répulsion. Sa tare de nègre-pie provoque les mêmes réactions négatives, les mêmes réticences que

---

[18] P. Lund et al., 'Variations in the Frequency of Albinism among Clans in the Venda Region of South Africa', *Journal of Medical Genetics*, 40 (2003), 823–38 (824).

[19] Stine Hellum-Braathen and Benedicte Ingstad, 'Albinism in Malawi: Knowledge and Belief from an African setting', *Disability and Society*, 21 (2006), 599–611 (600).

[20] Lund, 'Health and Education', 5.

les lépreux' (*Nègre blanc*, 235). This sense of repulsion at the albino body is echoed in Grainville's *Le Tyran éternel* when July reaches out to Alpha and then realises that it has been a long time since he had been touched (187). As Lund finds, in Zimbabwe it is believed that touching a person with albinism will result in the birth of a child with the condition.[21] The fear that pregnant women will be affected by touching, or even looking at a child with albinism, is echoed in Hanson's *Takadini* as Sekai and her baby seek refuge in the village which will eventually become their home: 'One man, whose young wife was pregnant, asked Chivero if he knew for sure what effect the sight of a *musope* would have on an unborn child' (66–7).[22]

People with albinism, like people with disabilities, were traditionally segregated in parts of sub-Saharan Africa. Today this segregation continues on a certain level as children with albinism are prevented from mixing with their peers for fear that the condition is contagious. A recent report in the Nigerian magazine *Newswatch* confirms the continued existence of such misconceptions, describing the experience of a student with the condition:

> At school many students didn't like to lend books, especially the notes given by their teachers. She couldn't copy directly from the board because of her vision impairment. Due to her colour and her sight problem, she had to be close to her teachers. 'Even if they didn't want to come close to me, I forced myself on them because I needed their lecture notes'.[23]

Describing the experiences of people with albinism in Tanzania Masha remarks that people will cross the road to avoid walking near them and children with the condition are prevented from playing with other children.[24] Some children with albinism are hidden away by their parents who are ashamed of them, and other parents believe that children with albinism

---

21 Ibid., 3.
22 *Musope* means that the child is born without a skin, that the child has albinism.
23 Onoja and Airahuobhor, 'Albinos – Tales of Mockery, Rejection', 49.
24 See Maryceline Masha, 'What Kind of Black are You?' *The Guardian, Tanzania* <http://www.vso.org.uk/publications/orbit/71/community.htm> [Accessed 30 June 2009].

are not as able as their normally pigmented counterparts so they are denied an education.[25] References can also be found in studies of albinism in Tanzania and Zimbabwe to the fact that if a person with albinism has touched food, it will not be eaten by anyone else.[26] This raises particular difficulties in societies in which food is often shared from a communal pot and in which not offering food to a visitor is unheard of. Similarly, in South Africa and Zimbabwe, after a person with albinism has drunk from a cup it will be broken, as though it has been contaminated.[27]

Not only do people with albinism face the refusal of others to shake hands and share taxis with them, but some even find their own family members keeping them at a distance.[28] One person with albinism describes reactions of friends and family members: 'My mother distances herself from me [...] I had girlfriends who preferred to quietly meet me without meeting me in public. You go to a party, they won't want to dance with you.'[29] Modern myths about albinism also abound in Africa today, adding to those beliefs surrounding albinism which have already been mentioned. The most striking of these is the belief that sexual intercourse with a woman with albinism can cure HIV AIDS.[30] Such responses to albinism appear ridiculous when its genetic provenance is recalled. However, the rooting of such misconceptions in traditional belief means that even when the cause of albinism is fully explained, an undercurrent of superstition remains.

25 Charlotte Baker, Patricia Lund, Julie Taylor and Richard Nyathi, 'Cultural and Literary Perspectives on the Myths Surrounding Albinism in Southern Africa', *Journal of African Cultural Studies*, 22.2 (2010), 175.
26 M. Bourdillon, *The Shona Peoples* (Gweru, Zimbabwe: Mambo Press, 1987), 57.
27 Baker et al. 'Cultural and Literary Perspectives on the Myths Surrounding Albinism in Southern Africa', 180.
28 Patricia Lund, 'Living with Albinism: A Study of Affected Adults in Zimbabwe', *Social Biology and Human Affairs*, 63.1 (1998), 3–9.
29 Rose Onoja and Andrew Airahuobhor, 'Albinos: Tales of Mockery, Rejection – Special Report', *Newswatch* (18 December 2006), 49–56 (56).
30 Patrick Nganzi and George Matenhodze, 'Disability and HIV AIDS'. Report commissioned by the International Corporation for Development. <http://www.asksource.info/pdf/32680_PRAdishiv_2004.pdf> [Accessed 8 February 2010].

Grainville illustrates perfectly the reluctance to accept the genetic explanation for albinism as Houphouët-Boigny reveals his horror at the revelation that Alpha is his son:

> J'assume une progéniture luxuriante. Mais un albinos! Mes gènes excluent cette tare, cette descendance larvaire. Il n'y a jamais eu d'albinos dans ma famille. Jamais. Nulle part. Depuis les origines. Point d'indétermination. Ce n'est pas notre genre. Par ma mère, une tribu de chefs akoués. Notre généalogie l'atteste. Mon père, soldat de Samori, le héros, le rebelle, le conquérant. (*Tyran*, 232)

Samate's father reacts in a similar way in Destremau's *Nègre blanc*, deciding that the child he sees in front of him cannot possible be his son: 'Il avait décidé que ce petit être ne serait pas son fils, qu'il n'était pas digne de figurer dans sa descendance' (47). The implication is that albinism is a stain on the reputation of the family, a sign of failure or weakness. Rather than admitting such genetic inheritance, the perceived failure is instead attributed to the mother of the child with albinism. In the case of Grainville's *Le Tyran éternel*, the responsibility is deemed to lie with Houphouët-Boigny's wife Masseni whom, in refusing to admit paternity, he implicitly accuses of infidelity.

Sassine's Maurice asks the young Milo, 'Petit, comment tu as fait pour être si blanc avec une mère noire?' (33), suggesting that Milo is in some way responsible for his whiteness. However, a journalist goes so far as to implicate Milo's mother, inciting Milo to exact his revenge:

> Ma dernière victime était une journaliste, très grande et belle et tout. [...] Elle était là pour un reportage, je lui ai montré une de tes photos, elle a commenté, 'Ta mère aurait dû tromper ton père'. Le lendemain, nous regardions une chute d'eau et je l'ai poussée. (45)

This statement is typical of the supposition that the birth of a child with albinism results from the mother's infidelity, an assumption that is raised several times and which, on each occasion, inspires Milo's vengeance. In Hanson's *Takadini*, the protagonist's mother is abandoned by her husband Kutukwa, who also suggests infidelity as the reason for the child's appearance: 'Tell me, woman, were you sharing your mat with some other man? And is this the punishment?' (28). Such assumptions of infidelity are common and Kutukwa's actions echo those of many fathers who desert the family at the birth of a baby with albinism, meaning that many grow up in single parent families.

Responsibility for the birth of a child with albinism is invariably placed with the mother, whether the explanation given for the birth is one of infidelity or of the mother having had intercourse during her period. Repeated references in the work of these writers are made to the birth of a child with albinism constituting a punishment of the mother or the parents for having committed an act considered unacceptable in the tribe or particular culture. In *Wirriyamu*, we learn that '[o]n croit ici que, quand une femme se lave la nuit sous un arbre, elle accouche d'un albinos' (184), and in *Le Tyran éternel*, Vieille Ada comments that 'les albinos naissent d'un amour monstrueux... un albinos ne peut naître que d'un désir terrifiant' (86).

The locating of culpability with the mother that is found in all four texts has serious consequences for both her and her child. Milo's mother abandons him shortly after his birth, Alpha is hidden away for fear of his father's reaction to him, and Condélo's mother is abandoned by all those who know her because her child resembles no other. Samate's mother Mbuya fears that the birth of her child is a punishment for a sin that she or her ancestors have committed:

> Elle jeta un nouveau regard furtif sur la petite bête qui respirait si vite, enfouie dans ses bras, sur ses seins gonflés. Aucun doute n'était permis: il présentait cette couleur iris pâle, avec des reflets roses, presque translucides [...] Mbuya fut envahie d'une immense et incontrôlable terreur. Bien que couverts de transpiration sous l'effet des efforts et de l'humidité ambiante, ses bras se mirent à frissonner. Elle eut soudain froid. Elle avait donc commis un lourd péché, elle ou ses ancêtres, et elle payait de cette façon la faute de son clan. (*Nègre blanc*, 29–30)

Thus, the birth of a child with albinism is established as a punishment for the misdemeanours not only of the mother, but of the family, and the stigma of albinism is passed on to all those associated with the person with the condition.

The Stigma of Albinism

Stigmatisation is a process by which particular human traits are deemed to be deviant, a process enacted in the literal or metaphorical marking apart of an individual who does not conform. This is facilitated when an individual is as clearly marked apart by physical difference as a person with albinism in Africa. In its most literal use, the term stigma refers to a mark or stain. This particular association is drawn from the Greek branding of slaves and criminals since the term stigma was used to refer to signs that were cut or burnt into the body to show that the bearer was a slave or a criminal; in Goffman's words, 'a blemished person, ritually polluted, to be avoided, especially in public places'.[31] Today the term stigma is attached to the disgrace itself as well as to the bodily evidence of it.

Goffman describes three types of stigma, the first of which are 'abominations of the body', that account for various physical deformities, of which albinism would be considered one.[32] Goffman contends that the visibility of a particular stigma is a crucial factor in determining whether an individual is to be stigmatised or not.[33] Although Goffman fails to discuss strategies of reaction other than that of passing and avoids the vital issue of resistance, his approach to the process of scapegoating is particularly relevant to the work of Destremau, Grainville and Sassine given the insistence of his theory of scapegoating on the process of marginalisation of certain individuals. Attributes such as skin colour and physical impairment provide visible evidence of stigma, so their bearer can be easily and immediately discredited. This process is evident in the four texts explored in this study, with the marking of the albino as deviant by stigmata such as skin and hair colour. Insistence on this 'marking apart' is particularly evident in Destremau's *Nègre blanc*, in which Samate is repeatedly described in terms

---

31   Erving Goffman, *Stigma – Notes on the Management of Spoiled Identity* (Harmondsworth: Penguin, 1963), 13.
32   Ibid., 14.
33   Ibid., 74.

Myth and Stereotype 71

of his difference. He is 'affublé dès la naissance de tares dont il souffre' (39), 'cette tare honteuse' (222), '[s]a tare de nègre-pie' (235) that makes him 'un être affligé d'une tare disgracieuse, qui l'exclut du genre humain' (236).

Goffman's argument that the more prominent the stigma, the more likely it is that it will affect the individual's social interactions, is clearly supported by literary representations of the prejudice suffered by people with albinism.[34] The consequences of such exclusion are illustrated in Sassine's *Mémoire d'une peau* by Milo's extreme behaviour, by his madness and his desire to kill, while for Grainville's Alpha, the insistence on his difference manifests itself in his choice to distance himself from society. Thus, the second stigma identified by Goffman – that of blemishes of individual character – is attached to the figure of the albino. The albino body is marked apart as the stigma of chromatic deviance is translated into social deviance and the perception that the chromatic deviance of albinism translates into social deviance becomes a reality as the consequences of the constant definition of an individual in terms of his difference manifests itself in extremes of behaviour.

It has become evident from my reading of these and other novels with albino characters that the perpetuation of stereotypes attached to the albino body promotes the stigmatisation of people with albinism and of individuals associated with that person. Nowhere is this more apparent than in Sassine's *Mémoire d'une peau* where the stigma of Milo's albinism is integral to his relationship with his mother. At the moment of his mother's revelation that she adopted him as a baby, Milo insists that she should not have kept him, because she could have had a 'normal' child. The consequences of Milo's mother Lucie having adopted a child with albinism are revealed as the narrative progresses and we learn that Milo's presence only added to '[sa] réputation de sorcière' (35). It is remarkable that Lucie

---

34 Goffman's distinguishes between discredited and discreditable stigma, using the term discredited to describe those who presume that their stigma is known about already or is immediately noticeable to others (as in the case of albinism). In contrast, the term discreditable is used by Goffman to describe those who believe that their stigma is not known to, or perceptible to others (as with epilepsy, for example). See Goffman, *Stigma*, 40.

agreed to adopt Milo in the first place, given the stigma attached to his albinism. Although not elaborated in the narrative, perhaps the fact that she is *métisse* and consequently marginalised allows her to empathise with the child. The same willingness of marginal characters to associate with people with albinism is seen in Rama's relationship with the adult Milo. Rama explains her situation:

> C'est Christian qui m'a libérée. Il m'a donné sa nationalité, son nom, sa confiance, son chéquier. Je viens d'un pays de merde de l'autre coté de l'Afrique… J'ai un frère au Canada, une sœur en France, une autre aux Etats-Unis, ma petite sœur avec nous. Nous avons été atomisés. Ma mere est toujours là-bas. (117)

Significantly, Rama is also an outsider in Guinea, which might explain her willingness to associate with Milo and her understanding of him. It is not only the mother of a child with albinism who shares the burden of the condition, but as Destremau's *Nègre blanc* suggests, the stigma is borne more widely:

> L'albinisme est une disgrâce pour le groupe, la marque d'une malédiction, la punition d'un péché qu'on admet devoir subir collectivement puisque les relations au sein de la tribu déterminent à tout moment la vie de chaque individu. (39)

Here, the presence of a person with albinism is interpreted as the sign of a misdemeanour for which the community must take collective responsibility.

Myths Surrounding Albinism

Describing the whiteness of albinism as 'la marque d'une malédiction' (*Nègre blanc*, 39), Destremau refers to the outward stigma or mark that designates the person with albinism as an emissary from the spirit world. Jennifer Kromberg notes that the colour white carries special significance in South Africa and that traditional doctors or diviners will often carry white beads, skins and cows' tails, or will sacrifice white goats.[35] White animals are sacred across cultures, symbols of purity, of the untouched and the untainted. In certain parts of Africa, only white animals are sacrificed, signifying that white is the colour of purity and the sacred, whereas elsewhere white is the colour associated with death, spirits, and evil.[36] Here we find that whiteness is not given the same connotations as it is in racial discourse, but instead signals a link to the spirit world, explaining Kromberg's speculation that the whiteness of people with albinism means that they are seen not as real mortals, but rather as spirits, or reincarnations of spirits.[37] As Blankenberg reminds us, it is important to recognise that these perceptions are not ancient folklore, taken with a grain of salt in contemporary Africa, but are very much believed in and acted on to this day.[38] In her study of African realism and the sub-Saharan African novel, Claire Dehon also notes: 'En Afrique subsaharienne, les gens n'ont pas abandonné d'anciennes façons de penser ou de voir le monde: l'invisible et le visible coexistent, le surnaturel se manifeste aujourd'hui encore sans que l'homme puisse toujours prévenir ses interventions.'[39]

Throughout the world, myths function to account for phenomena which are out of the ordinary, or which cannot be explained in other terms, fulfilling a fundamental human need to make sense of the world. The beliefs surrounding albinism are often found to compensate for such a lack of knowledge. Despite the wealth of research and documentation on the genetic nature of albinism, a failure to communicate this has resulted in the continued misunderstanding that surrounds the condition. In their

---

35   Jennifer Kromberg, 'Albinism in the South African Negro: Attitudes and the Death Myth', *Birth Defects: Original Article Series*, 28 (1988), 159–66.

36   Françoise Parent Ugochukwu, 'The Devil's Colors: A Comparative Study of French and Nigerian Folktales', *Oral Tradition*, 21 (2007), 1–18.

37   Kromberg, 'Albinism in the South African Negro', 162. Grainville describes Whites in similar terms in his 1978 novel *Les Flamboyants*, where they are described as, 'les diables [...] pour nous les nègres, ils sont blancs comme de la neige'. Patrick Grainville, *Les Flamboyants* (Paris: Poche, 1978), 36.

38   Ibid., 14.

39   Claire L. Dehon, *Le Réalisme africain: le roman francophone en Afrique subsaharienne* (Paris: L'Harmattan, 2002), 16.

study of albinism in Malawi, Hellum-Braathen and Ingstad found that the parents of people with albinism had not been given an adequate explanation as to the cause of their child's condition.[40] Even when the genetic explanation for albinism is accepted, it often runs parallel to existing beliefs. As Blankenberg elucidates, 'elements which through a Western derived logic ought to cancel each other out, often in reality do not: inyangas and medical clinics are consulted simultaneously; skins and suits are worn next to each other'.[41]

In their study of albinism in South America, Jeambrun and Sergent comment:

> Les sociétés répondent différemment à l'albinos. Les unes réagissent très fortement à la présence des albinos en leur sein: c'est le cas de l'Afrique sub-saharienne, qui, en de nombreux cas, mythifie ses albinos, ou leur confère des fonctions sacerdotales, ou les sacrifie.[42]

While some myths are held continent- and world-wide, for various reasons others are restricted to particular locations. Characters with albinism appear in myths and oral tales throughout Africa, one example being the albino created in error by Obatala, the Yoruba God of Creation. Wole Soyinka describes how 'Obatala, moulder of men, fell [...] to the fumes of wine; his craftsman's fingers lost their control and he moulded cripples, albinos, the blind and other deformed.'[43] The figure of the albino appears too in the Dogon myth in which Yasigui gives birth to a child with albinism instead of the expected twins, a punishment for transgressing tribal rules. The Aandonga, in the south of Angola, tell of the albino being an ogre (*esisi*) while the Mayombe of the Congo believe them to be spirit children and observe particular ceremonies on the birth of a person with albinism. Albinos also appear in the Maori myth *Ko Mutalau mo Matuku-hifi* and there frequent references to albino animals are found in the mythology of Native American Indians.

40 Hellum-Braathen and Ingstad, 'Albinism in Malawi', 603.
41 Blankenberg, 'That Rare and Random Tribe', 12.
42 Jeambrun and Sergent, *Les Enfants de la lune*, 213.
43 Wole Soyinka, *Myth, Literature and the African World* (Cambridge: Canto, 1976), 159.

Myth and Stereotype

The association of albinism with the moon is frequently made in fictional writing, and we find two examples in *Le Tyran éternel* as Grainville's Tanella, President of the Writers' Union, attributes the adjectives 'lunaire et chaotique' (26) to the albino. Later, the narrator considers the relationship between the figure of the albino, the moon and the world of the dead:

> Parce qu'on le détestait lui, qu'on s'écartait de lui, qu'il dégoûtait, qu'il faisait peur, qu'il semblait revenir de la Lune et de la mort, qu'il vous rendait coupable. (186)

The description of people with albinism as 'les enfants de la lune' by the San Blas Indians refers to the common belief that they can only be seen by night, which is perpetuated by the avoidance of the sunlight by people with albinism because it can be so harmful to their skin. However, it is also an interesting collocation given the link between women and the moon in lunar myths of fertility, considering the insistence on the guilt that rests with the mother upon the birth of a child with the albinism. Since the moon is frequently linked to madness – the word 'lunatic' being derived from the Latin *luna* – Milo's comment in *Mémoire d'une peau* that people with albinism 'préfèrent la nuit à la lumière...' (134) is of particular significance, since his madness manifests itself by night, when the majority of his crimes take place.

The San Blas call people with albinism 'moon-children' not only because they avoid the sun, but because it is believed that they can see in the dark.[44] The same ability is attributed to Samate in Destremau's *Nègre blanc*:

> On disait d'eux qu'ils portaient le mauvais œil, justement parce qu'ils pouvaient voir la nuit, non seulement les choses mais surtout les forfaits qu'accomplissaient les êtres humains à l'abri de l'obscurité, de même que ce qu'ils concoctaient au tréfonds de leurs âmes. Cette capacité extranaturelle, ces pouvoirs extralucides accordés par la divinité à ces humains extraordinaires, qu'on disait être les auxiliaires des divinités mauvaises acharnées à la perte des hommes, terrifiaient tout le monde, sauf leur entourage immédiat. (30)

---

44 Wan, 'Orange in a World of Apples', 277.

Not only are people with albinism supposed to be able to see by night, but their apparent ability to see into the depths of the souls of others is just one of many mystical powers ascribed to them.

The association of albinism with death is returned to time and again, in the work of Grainville in particular, as DjeDje describes people with albinism as 'the living dead' and Houphouët-Boigny refers to Alpha as a walking corpse. In *Wirriyamu* too, the albino becomes a phantasmal, spectral figure, an image compounded by his cadaverous, colourless skin, which Kabalango describes as the colour of a shroud (*Wirriyamu*, 60). Houphouët-Boigny asserts: '[l'albinos] porte mort. Il revient des morts. Il n'a jamais quitté la mort. Il n'a jamais opéré le partage. Il est un entre-deux détestable' (*Tyran*, 116), expressing the idea of the intermediary nature of the albino that is a common motif in fictional writing. In a recent study of albinism in sub-Saharan Africa, Aquaron et al. describe the status of the albino:

> Considéré comme un authentique 'africain blanc', l'albinos n'en reste pas moins ressenti comme appartenant à un monde magique qui fait de lui une créature humaine intermédiaire inachevée, demi homme – demi dieu, dotée des pouvoirs innés à partir desquels il décide de faire du bien et du mal.[45]

In their study of Soyinka's *The Interpreters*, in which the albino character Lazarus appears, Karen and Morell also refer to the notion of the *revenant*, positioned between two worlds: 'L'albinos, en effet, est une créature crépusculaire qui n'appartient pas entièrement à notre monde; c'est un symbole physique de la région des transitions.'[46] Karen and Morell's description recalls Blankenberg's explanation of the albino as an emissary from the spirit world, once again a reference to the intermediary position of the albino, between the living and the dead, playing a role in both, yet belonging to neither.

---

45 Robert Aquaron, Médard Djatou, L. Kamdem, 'Aspects socioculturels des albinos en Afrique Noire: des mutilations et crimes rituels perpétrés en Afrique de l'Est (Burundi et Tanzanie)', *Médicine Tropicale* 69.5 (2009) 449–53 (449).
46 Edward Karen and L. Morell, *Person, Achebe, Awoonor and Soyinka* (Seattle, Institute for Comparative Foreign Areas Studies, 1975) cited in Chevrier, *Williams Sassine: écrivain de la marginalité*, 273.

Myth and Stereotype

In death, people with albinism are not only set apart spiritually, but also physically. In some parts of Africa, they are buried by night, their graves placed at a distance from the usual burial grounds. In the same way, in Destremau's *Nègre blanc*, Mbuya recalls having heard that the bodies of infants are buried away from other graves: 'N'étant pas considéré comme déjà entré dans le monde réel des vivants, le corps du nourrisson n'a pas plus de valeur que celui d'un animal domestique et est enterré à part, loin du cimetière traditionnel' (38). The devalued body of the albino is equated with that of the *nourrisson* or a domestic animal. However, it is impossible to generalise when speaking of the beliefs surrounding the death of a person with albinism. For example, Djatou notes that:

> Les Bakweri enterrent les albinos sous les grandes racines d'un arbre (baobab) appelé 'bouma'. Cet arbre-talisman est reconnu pour sa sollicitation par les sorciers et les génies. Une fois sous les racines de cet arbre, la dépouille de l'albinos est recouverte de feuilles de banane et il est fortement pensé qu'après trois jours, cette dépouille disparaît. Ce qui veut dire que le défunt a rejoint le monde des esprits.[47]

Despite the changes that have taken place in rural Cameroon with the introduction of coffins and cemeteries in modern burials, the Bakweri continue to plant a Bouma sapling on the grave of a person with albinism as a mark of respect.

Sacrifice

In *Nègre blanc*, Destremau portrays the killing of disabled children as a secretive act that is carried out discreetly:

> Dès qu'une naissance anormale est signalée, et Dieu sait que les informations courent vite dans la tribu, les vieilles femmes se réunissent et prennent une décision qui souvent se résume à la mort afin de ne pas alourdir la charge du clan. (37–8)

---

47   Djatou, unpublished doctoral study, 56–7.

As Destremau's novel indicates, the decision as to whether or not a child is to live is often in the hands of very influential older women. In Hanson's novel *Takadini*, the midwives look closely at the child they have delivered: 'Newly born infants are usually much lighter in complexion than their parents. However, even in the dim firelight this baby seemed *too light*' (*Takadini*, 12). The midwife Ambuya Tukai's initial reaction is to suggest that because the baby is *musope* it must be destroyed, but her assistant Ambuya Sungu suggests that Sekai should be allowed to experience the joy of motherhood, if only for a few hours. This resolution to allow the child to live is decisive for Takadini and his mother Sekai. However, later in the narrative, we learn that the same belief is held in the village to which Sekai escapes with her child: 'We all know the tradition of our forefathers throughout the land, in every clan and village. Such children must be killed; deformed children must be killed; and one of twins must be destroyed' (*Takadini*, 57).

In direct contrast to this clandestine act of infanticide, the sacrifice of people with albinism in Destremau's *Nègre blanc* is portrayed as a symbolic, shared act. Describing the sacrifice of a baby with the condition, Mbuya recalls a ritual in which the child is lifted by the *nganga* towards the sky against a background of incantations before he is projected into the torrid waters of the river. Recalling the act later, Mbuya experiences a passing sense of guilt that she did nothing at the time, but decides that this remorse is a result of the trauma she has suffered in discovering that her child has albinism. However, the memory leads her to reflect on the possibility that her own baby might meet the same fate, motivating her to leave the village, determining the course of her life and that of her child Samate.

Sassine's Milo perfunctorily drops the comment into conversation: 'Nous servons de sacrifices dans certaines régions d'Afrique' (*Mémoire*, 133). However, the grave significance of these words is exposed in *Wirriyamu* as Sassine focuses on the last days of Condélo's life, evoking the young man's fear and naivety as he is pursued in the belief that the blood of the albino brings luck. Ritual sacrifice means that the previously devalued albino body takes on significance in death. The blood of the albino is suddenly endowed with value: 'Le sang de l'albinos est le meilleur garant pour une rapide et brillante réussite' (82). In the same way, disgust at the whiteness of albino skin is replaced by awe as the symbolism of whiteness is interpreted as a

Myth and Stereotype

sign that the person with albinism is a messenger from the spirit world. Grainville's Masseni confirms that in the act of human sacrifice the albino body gains value: 'Si les albinos ont été sacrifiés, c'est parce qu'ils rendaient les sacrifices efficaces. Le sorcier, loin d'insister sur la honte attachée aux albinos, a souligné leur puissance' (*Tyran*, 230).

One passage in Sassine's *Wirriyamu* in particular demonstrates the value placed on the sacrificed albino body, which is shared out in a manner that recalls the act of Holy Communion:

> Lorsque j'étais tout petit, mon père fit venir un jour, devant notre case, un albinos ligoté. Deux nuits durant, nous avons tous dansé de joie. La troisième nuit, en ma présence et avec application, il égorgea l'albinos au-dessus d'une énorme calebasse. Ensuite il dépeça le corps et le partagea entre tous nos villageois. Certains morceaux furent bien ficelés et expédiés à ses meilleurs amis. Après, il me lava le visage de son sang et fit de même pour tous mes autres frères. Il s'en enduisit lui-même la figure et les bras avant d'en offrir au fétiche de la famille. Je grandis avec la tranquille et sereine assurance d'être désormais protégé du mauvais sort. (81)

Overtly religious references such as this are by no means incidental in Sassine's work. As Chevrier observes, in *Wirriyamu* and in Sassine's other fictional work, we see the man who attentively read the Christian Bible and studied the Koran encounter the boy who cannot forget the tales he heard during his childhood in Kankan.[48] Indeed, the above quotation could equally be read as an example of ritual human sacrifice and cannibalism.

The quotation also brings to mind the meeting and conflict of African traditional beliefs and Western religion that runs through Sassine's *Wirriyamu* as well as Grainville's *Le Tyran éternel*. Both novels refer back to a past in which traditional beliefs were practised, including that of ritual human sacrifice. Grainville's Houphouët-Boigny remembers Yamoussoukro, 'mon village natal où, enfant, avant ma conversion, j'assistais encore à des sacrifices' (*Tyran*, 11), and admits that his Christianity is bound up with paganism and an African spirituality that has not completely abandoned its traditions of myth, polygamy and sacrifice. In Sassine's *Wirriyamu*, we find another individual who embodies what Chevrier terms 'un double

---

48 Chevrier, *Williams Sassine: écrivain de la marginalité*, 136.

système spirituel'.[49] Père Fidel, the priest of Wirriyamu, is haunted by his inability to choose between traditional beliefs and the Christianity to which he was converted. Chevrier describes him as:

> Ce païen converti au christianisme, hanté par ses fantasmes sexuels et taraudé par la mauvaise conscience, apparaît en effet comme l'une des figures les plus douloureuses du roman, en raison précisément de son appartenance à un double système spirituel, et de son incapacité foncière à opter pour l'une ou l'autre voie.[50]

Beneath the references to a time when human sacrifice was practiced in Africa and the meeting and conflict of these beliefs with Western religion, an undertone of uncertainty runs through *Wirriyamu*. Sacrifice in the belief that the blood of the albino has certain powers is portrayed as a betrayal, the result of a fabrication of beliefs of which he is ultimately a victim. The first suggestion of this occurs early in the narrative: 'La tradition s'était donc établie, sans effort et sans contestation, tout aussi naturelle que le jour et la nuit, la souffrance et le plaisir. Personne ne savait quel âge elle avait, d'où elle provenait' (40). This suggestion is developed by Kabalango, elderly and terminally ill, who when we first meet him is returning to his village to die. Later, as he attempts to unearth the foundations of the belief that the blood of the albino brings health and success, Kabalango discovers that 'elle avait été ou introduite ou encouragée par les Portugais car l'un de leurs premiers administrateurs, il y a de cela très longtemps, assiégé par une de nos tribus en révolte, ne dut sa survie qu'au sang d'un albinos' (82).

As Tanella explains in *Le Tyran éternel*, all societies invent scapegoats onto which they project their fears and guilt. In *Wirriyamu* in particular, the need to project problems onto an individual who can be clearly identified as different or marginal is clear. When this process is considered in terms of René Girard's theory of scapegoating it becomes clear why the figure of the albino should be a victim of such beliefs.[51] Girard identifies the particular moment at which the need for a scapegoat is most pressing

---

49   Ibid., 47.
50   Idem.
51   René Girard, *Le Bouc emissaire* (Paris: Grasset, 1982).

as being a point in time at which there is a collapse of order. In *Wirriyamu*, this 'order' is represented by the colonial rule of the Portuguese, which at the time of the action is breaking down into anarchy. The search for a scapegoat, against whom the community will unite, leads to the penultimate stage in which violence results in the death of the victim, after which calm will descend. Girard suggests that over time, discord will reappear, so it becomes necessary to recapture a sense of peace. The final step in the process is the ritual of sacrifice, a practice of substitution that functions as a re-enactment of the original murder with an innocent victim as a substitute sacrifice. Scapegoating, like stereotyping, is exposed as a process by which an individual or group is discredited, or rendered 'different' in order to satisfy the needs of others.

According to Girard, the scapegoat is the key component of any sacrifice.[52] A sacrificial substitute is selected by the group, because killing the individual who is actually responsible for the escalation of violence would only elicit and encourage further violence. In Sassine's *Wirriyamu*, this scapegoat is the figure of the albino Condélo, who is pursued to his death. Girard suggests that the scapegoat must both resemble and differ considerably from the subject it replaces. In a society founded upon the hierarchy of white over black, the albino seems the obvious target in the colonial society of Wirriyamu. The ambiguous characteristics of the sacrificial substitute ensure that because of its similarity to the instigator of the unrest, the violence is actually contained. On the other hand, the dissimilarity of the sacrificial substitute to the original subject ensures that no further escalation of violence results after the sacrifice is performed. Through this process, the sacrificial substitute provides a space for and delimits violence by providing a legitimate outlet for it.

Examples of vilification and blame are evident in all four fictional texts explored in *Enduring Negativity* and expose the necessity of discrediting certain sections of the population in order to maintain the stability of others. This in itself belies the near-impossibility of breaking down stereotypes. The very nature of the stereotype means that, in destroying one, another

---

52   Ibid., 28.

must necessarily be formed in its place in order to maintain the established hierarchy. Hence, resistance to stereotypes is often self-defeating, although there are many ways in which they can be resisted or challenged. If one stereotype must necessarily be replaced by another, then the most positive outcome would be the transformation of negative stereotypes into more positive ones. The creation of countertypes offers the possibility of celebrating those attributes previously considered in a negative way. The countertype is a positive stereotype that evolves from the attempt to replace a negative stereotype that has been applied to a specific group of people.

In the acting out and confirmation of stereotypes, it is possible for the stereotyped individual to take account of his or her perceived difference and to act upon it. Milo, for example, identifies the albino with the animal in need of protection in his encouragement of the charity of philanthropic women. In so doing, he reveals how easily the stereotypes of albinism can be manipulated in his favour and simultaneously exposes the self-interest of the women:

> Au fond de la boîte, je remarquai les inévitables touristes, hommes en cabots, avec chemises en fleurs, leurs femmes grimmées en mannequins boudinés, genre mammouth ou petites folles décontractées et remuantes prêtes à ôter leur tee-shirt du Prisunic, jusqu'à leur peau qui leur faisait mal parce qu'elles ne grillaient pas assez vite au soleile de leur Afrique [...] Je leur apprenais à s'émouvoir sur ma condition. Elles rêvaient alors d'une société protectrice des albinos, une autre SPA et se voyaient déjà célèbres comme Brigitte Bardot. (*Mémoire*, 73–4)

An alternative means of breaking down stereotypes is suggested by Rosello, who proposes that declining a stereotype is a way of depriving it of its harmful potential by highlighting its very nature.[53] In his use of humour, for example, Sassine reveals the rhetoric of stereotyping as superficial discourse. With the fact of his albinism in mind, Milo remarks that he has little more chance of finding love than of becoming the next Pope (18). A series of such self-referential comments occur throughout *Mémoire d'une peau*. On another occasion, Milo asks himself: 'Milo Kan, qu'est-ce que tu

---

53   Rosello, *Declining the Stereotype*, 11.

as à te reprocher mon petit vieux? Accroche-toi au présent. Les idées ne te disent plus grand-chose. Tu ne crois qu'aux corps ?' (8). The obvious irony here is that there is no escape from the reality of his albino body. Although humorous on the surface, the significance of Milo's comments is profound and the sensitivity of the subject is masked in wit. Whether the stereotype is declined through ironic repetition, the distortion of language or the overt use of puns, the purpose is the same; that is, to challenge stereotypes and the process by which they are created.

The fine line between the presence of active stereotypes and the fictional representation of stereotypes is revealed as problematic for writers and for critics attempting to distinguish between the two. Jan Nederveen Pieterse contends that stereotypes function as self-fulfilling prophecies, a process by which 'the targets of stereotyping are manoeuvred into certain roles so that a vicious circle develops in which reality seems to endorse the stereotype'.[54] Just as stereotypes and reality are bound up, stereotypes and representation are intimately linked, since stereotyping is a process of representation, and representation is in turn a process of stereotyping. Novels expressly written in reaction to stereotypes frequently include a number of digressions which specifically refute major misconceptions. The characters often display only those traits that counteract the pejorative ones that are associated with the stereotype, attempting to posit substitute positive stereotypes for the more familiar negative ones.

Although Destremau, Grainville and Sassine portray their protagonists as individuals, the novels fail to escape the fact of stereotyping altogether. Only fictional writing that presents people with albinism as individuals and not in terms of the traits that link them with other people with the condition or posit them as representative can truly move beyond stereotypes. However, the question of visibility then becomes a pertinent one, for if people with albinism are not described as such, is the condition not at risk of being written over? The novels are in many ways typical of stereotypical representations of albinism, presenting the figure of the albino as

---

54 Jan Nederveen-Pieterse, *White on Black: Images of Africa and Blacks in Western Popular Culture* (New Haven: Yale University Press, 1992), x.

deviant and in turn signalling conventional and traditional claims to the superiority of bodily, racial and sexual forms that represent the illusion of normality. Many of the stereotypes of albinism that occur in the work of Destremau, Grainville and Sassine are deliberate, but the stereotypical language they employ less so. For, as we have already mentioned, bound up in the language of race and colour, of ability and disability, are references that are inescapable.

The stigma of albinism and the process of categorisation through stereotyping clearly underlie the work of Destremau, Grainville and Sassine, and although there has been some suggestion by critics that the act of stereotyping has certain positive functions, the over-ridingly negative impact of the stereotype upon the stereotyped individual is undeniable. The problematic nature of stereotypes is expressed by Bhabha, who critiques the 'limiting and traditional reliance on the stereotype as offering, at any one time, a secure point of identification'.[55] He argues instead that the stereotype is 'a complex, ambivalent, contradictory mode of representation, as anxious as it is assertive'.[56] The multifarious nature and ambivalence of stereotypes problematise the possibility of challenging them. Although this near-impossibility of breaking down stereotypes has been addressed by critics, and in spite of the many suggestions as to how they can be challenged from within, there appears to be a universal acceptance that the fact of stereotyping must first be recognised in order to confront it. For this reason, a world without stereotypes seems unthinkable.

The difficulties that result for the stereotyped or stigmatised individual attempting to define an identity are central to the novels explored here, and although the writers approach the process of stereotyping from different standpoints, people with albinism remain vulnerable to the imposition of a fabricated identity. Identity has long been imposed onto the albino body in the form of myths, beliefs and stereotypes, and despite the changing values attributed to it; the consequence of imposing meaning onto the body is to deny individuality. It has become clear that the tendency is to

---

55 Bhabha, 'The Other Question', 69–70.
56 Ibid., 70.

homogenise people with albinism, to view the individual as representative of all people with the condition in the same way that the African individual was considered representative of all Africans under colonisation. It is not simply the act of stereotyping that is of interest here, but the process of subjectification which results, for it denies individuality. It is with this in mind that the following chapter will address issues of inclusion and exclusion, questioning the value placed on certain attributes over others and the significance attached to them.

CHAPTER 3

Inclusion and Exclusion

The notion of difference to which Destremau, Grainville and Sassine return frequently is evidentiary of the ways in which power comes to be inscribed. It raises questions with regard to relations of inequality and the manner in which differences are expressed among individuals, as well as between and within different groups. The preceding chapter explored the assertion and control of difference through stereotyping, an act that is frequently based on false assumptions or upon impression without direct experience. Stereotyping ascribes traits to individuals or groups and involves suppositions of characteristics thought to be common in an act of homogenisation. Operating as an apparatus of exclusion that serves to protect the 'norm', the stereotype asserts difference as deviance, rather than positing difference more positively as a mark of individuality. This chapter will explore further the need to exclude people with albinism – physically, socially or psychologically – and the ubiquitous consequences of such exclusion. The construction of boundaries, physical and metaphorical, imagined and constructed, will be examined, as will the means and consequences of imposing such limits. The chapter will then go on to explore the need to 'belong' and the possibility of inclusion of people with albinism, while considering the importance of a sense of belonging and acceptance for the marginalised individual.

Manuel Castells argues that 'It is easy to agree on the fact that [...] all identities are socially constructed. The real issue is how, from what, by whom and for what.'[1] The construction of boundaries and the marking of difference are integral to the defining of albino identity, for the marginality of people with albinism is shaped in terms of what is perceived

---

1   Manuel Castells, *The Power of Identity* (London: Blackwell, 1997), 7.

to be lacking or inadequate in that individual and by their failure to meet the criteria of acceptability. Bhabha opens *The Location of Culture* with a quote from Heidegger: 'A boundary is not that at which something stops but, as the Greeks recognised, the boundary is that from which *something begins its presencing*.'² As Heidegger acknowledges, the construction of the boundary emerges as a means of social control that is closely related to the organisation of power in society. Boundaries function both to protect and to differentiate, at once imposing and resisting difference, dictating the inclusion of certain individuals and the exclusion of others. In this chapter I will explore the ways in which the novels of Destremau, Grainville and Sassine reveal that the straddling of boundaries, whether of race, sexuality, ability, disability (or more than one of these in the case of people with albinism) results in a complication of identity and renders belonging problematic.

Forms of Exclusion

The themes of inclusion and exclusion, the consequence of the construction of social and cultural boundaries, and the imposition of limits are central to Destremau and Grainville's novels in particular. The contiguous fear of and fascination with what lies beyond the boundary or outside the limits reveals the need to contain and to delimit the deviant or the threatening, excluding it from the realm of acceptance. Thus, exclusion must be recognised as a social construction and not a natural phenomenon, for the form it takes – and the very process of its manifestation – is dependent upon its frame of reference. Exclusion occurs in many guises and operates on many different levels. As I will show in this chapter, exclusion might take the form of the physical segregation of a stigmatised individual, or if the exclusion is not physical, it occurs in the form of the alienation of an individual

---

2   Martin Heidegger, 'Building, Dwelling, Thinking', cited in Bhabha, *The Location of Culture*, 1.

within a group, effected by a constant reinforcing of his or her difference. Alternately, an individual might choose to distance him or herself from a society that threatens his or her well-being or sense of identity. Thus it becomes evident that exclusion is relative and relational, and involves more than just those individuals to whom it ostensibly refers.

Of all these means of exclusion, enforced physical expulsion from society operates most overtly in the novels in question. Destremau's Mbuya is forced to escape her village to take refuge in the savannah with her child, an event that later comes to be seen by the boy in terms of a forced expulsion: 'Moi, j'ai été exclu de ma tribu par la fuite de ma mère pour me sauver la vie' (*Nègre blanc*, 230). Sassine's Condélo is also driven from his birthplace in the village of Wirriyamu to seek refuge in the forest, 'la tête de l'albinos mise à prix' (*Wirriyamu*, 43).[3] These places are represented as spaces of retreat and Samate's later visits to the forest as a teenager are clearly presented as a return to his roots '[il] se replonge dans son élément originel' (*Nègre blanc*, 247). Similarly, the forest is represented as a space of security for Grainville's Alpha when he is excluded from his birthplace by the tyrannical Houphouët-Boigny, expelled because there is no space for the albino within the constructed boundaries of Yamoussoukro.

The novels demonstrate that the physical exclusion of people with albinism results from the construction of difference as a result of stereotypes, myths or religious beliefs. The 'otherness' of albinism is presented as all-defining, or at the most extreme, all-negating for the protagonists. As Milo recognises, 'Pour eux, j'étais un invisible, un rien' (*Mémoire*, 14). Likewise, in Sassine's *Wirriyamu*, a young child witnessing Condélo's suffering asks his father why the boy is being treated like an animal and is told by his father: 'Chacun a ses problèmes, mon enfant… ça ne nous regarde pas' (*Wirriyamu*, 17). The man's indifference is a constituent part of a process of ostracism and rejection which results not only in the social isolation of the person with albinism, but which often provokes their social exclusion too. The exclusion of the albino protagonists is created and maintained through the assertion of difference, and as a result their non-belonging is affirmed.

3   As the following chapter will make clear, the significance of the portrayal of the forest or the savannah as a space of sanctuary for the albino characters cannot be overlooked.

Researchers and theorists in the area of social exclusion and rejection acknowledge that such aversive behaviours as ostracism threaten a fundamental need to belong.[4] In his memoir, *Too White to be Black and Too Black to be White*, Edwards recalls the fear he faced every day as he grew up: 'Usually I had no idea what to expect when I stepped out of my front door each day. There were mostly bad experiences and sadly I had no defense against the negativism. I was swamped by it.'[5] Such victimisation is found in Sassine's *Wirriyamu*, in which we learn of the mistreatment suffered by Condélo at school as Vasconcelos tells of what he witnessed:

> Parfois, lorsque les cris des enfants me dérangeaient, je passais la tête au dessus de la clôture et, presque toujours, je l'apercevais acculé à un arbre, son pagne cachant sa figure pour refuser de voir les mottes de boue que lui lançaient, en hurlant de joie quand ils l'atteignaient, les autres petits. Après, il se dénudait d'un air indifférent et allait se laver. (*Wirriyamu*, 50)

Condélo is excluded from his peer group and made a victim throughout his life. The hatred felt towards this visibly different child manifests itself in the physical form of bullying to which he is evidently accustomed, as his reaction is simply to walk away and wash himself. Condélo's experiences echo those of pupils with albinism in mainstream schools in contemporary sub-Saharan Africa, who encounter problems of name-calling, bullying and physical victimisation. Samate and Milo find that teachers as well as students can be the source of mockery and derision. Destremau's Samate is described as solitary, with few friends other than his cousins. A lack of understanding of his condition and a failure to recognise the young boy's difference as anything other than negative renders the relationship between him and his peers a very superficial one. In this way, in *Nègre blanc* Destremau portrays Samate's sense of alienation and highlights the profound consequences of such social isolation for people with albinism.

---

4   Over the last decade there has been increased interest in the related social phenomena of ostracism, exclusion and rejection. See for example, Kipling Williams, *Ostracism: The Power of Silence* (New York: Guilford Press, 2002) and William Von Hippel, *The Social Outcast: Ostracism, Social Exclusion, Rejection, and Bullying* (New York: Taylor and Francis, 2005).

5   Edwards, *Too White to be Black and Too Black to be White*, 42.

The figure of the albino is consistently portrayed in literary representation as something other than normal, outside of culturally accepted boundaries and, for reasons which have already been addressed in Chapter 2, as an individual whose very presence is perceived to represent a threat. As Grainville's Alpha recalls, 'On m'a fait sentir dans mon enfance que mon existence même était un scandale, constituait une menace' (*Tyran éternel*, 172). Yet, for Destremau's Samate, no such early realisation is possible given his sheltered upbringing; a factor that perhaps heightens the consequences of this ostracism when it does eventually occur. Distanced from the outside world, Samate is ignorant of the implications of his albinism and it is only when he reaches his adoptive father's country of Rhodesia that he comes to realise the consequences of his albinism.

Williams notes that ostracism is a powerful metaphor for social death. Targets of ostracism become socially invisible when excluded from society and in this sense, he argues, they cease to exist.[6] Throughout the secondary literature on albinism copious references to the social problems faced by people with albinism are found, confirming the validity of the portrayal of such exclusion in literary representation. Examples given range from ostracism to overt bullying, including prejudicial treatment in every aspect of life, from access to education and employment to the availability of healthcare. Even if a child with albinism is sent to school, Agnès Wuthrich notes that these children often have difficulty in integrating. Not only are they prevented from participating by their visual disability, but also by the prejudices that they encounter.[7] Therefore, the exclusion of an individual within society is portrayed as equally damaging as his or her physical removal from it. It is a denial of that individual's existence, which is founded on the whiteness that marks him or her apart in black Africa. In the negation of an already fragile identity the consequences of such exclusion are revealed as profound.

The novels of Destremau, Grainville and Sassine suggest that the consequences of enforced exclusion from social intercourse are not very different from those resulting from the spontaneous decision of an individual to

---

6   Williams, *Ostracism*, 124.
7   Agnès Wuthrich, 'Un espoir pour les hommes sans couleur'. *Le Temps du Monde*, 18 novembre 2000 <http://www.letemps.ch/tour/reportages/etape16/jour322.html> [Accessed 3 August 2009].

distance him or herself from society. However, it is important to distinguish such voluntary exit from coerced or involuntary expulsion. In the case of an elective distancing from society, the inference is that the individual has made a deliberate choice to dissociate him or herself, whatever the reasons for that decision. The retreat of Grainville's protagonist is portrayed as a form of self-protection:

> J'ai dû changer de campement et de compagnons de travail. Et là, au bout de quelques mois, un type m'a fait sentir que j'étais différent. Il a convaincu les autres que je leur portais malheur. J'ai définitivement disparu dans la forêt. (*Tyran*, 221)

Such forms of physical distancing place the agency with the individual who breaks away from society and Alpha's solution is to 'disappear', in retreat from all that marks him as different. Yet, ironically, the consequences of this withdrawal from society serve only to confirm his deviance, for as the previous chapter revealed, every opportunity is taken to discredit the albino in the constitution and encouragement of myths and stereotypes that ultimately function to preserve his exclusion. The fact that Alpha has deliberately distanced himself gives the tyrannical leader the ideal opportunity to repudiate the very existence of the albino and Alpha's exclusion is confirmed. He becomes 'un bel albinos solitaire' (86), 'un type condamné à se planquer, à errer' (88). Alpha's distancing of himself from the city of Yamoussoukro serves only to encourage the dictatorial Houphouët-Boigny's continued assertion of the albino's non-belonging, which in turn allows him to protect his own precarious position.

Writers and critics have long noted that the loss of social bonds can unleash the most profound forms of human pain and suffering, and this is clearly reflected in Destremau's *Nègre blanc*. It is only as the young Samate tells his adoptive father Mafavuca of his escape from his native village that the older man realises the lasting consequences of the boy's separation from his tribe:

> Mafavuca est plus ému qu'il n'y paraît. La détermination de l'enfant de conserver ses liens intimes avec ses ancêtres en dépit de la rupture, du reniement et de l'isolement le touche. La bravoure de Samate dans plusieurs occasions s'explique, car s'il souhaite se montrer digne de la lignée à laquelle il appartient, il veut autant fourbir son image vis-à-vis de son père adoptif, et avant tout se situer par rapport à lui-même. (230–1)

Paradoxically, Samate's social exclusion only increases his desire for tribal and familial inclusion. Even as an adult in Rhodesia, despite his perfect mastery of the English language, he prefers to express himself in his native tongue. The sense of impending betrayal that he feels at abandoning his native language indicates his need to maintain links with the tribe despite his early separation from them. Although he longs to return to the forest, a place he associates with freedom, Samate realises that he cannot disclose this to his adoptive father, his only confidant, for fear of appearing ungrateful:

> Par bonté et amour pour ce Blanc si dévoué à sa cause, Samate préfère se taire et endurer seul ses tourments. Il doute cependant que le temps pourra les effacer comme il fait disparaître les trâces de sentiers dans la forêt, mais il se prépare à une existence de frustration dans le seul but de ne pas peiner son père adoptif, si vénéré et admiré. (260)

Social Exile

The consequences of exclusion are portrayed as equally profound for Sassine's Milo who, despite his extreme and anti-social behaviour, invites a degree of empathy when he comments: 'Mon passé ne me permet pas d'avoir confiance longtemps dans les autres' (*Mémoire*, 60). In contrast to Alpha, Condélo and Samate's physical expulsion from society, Milo's exclusion takes the form of social exile within society. Milo deliberately distances himself from a society in which he fails to fit. His is an affirmation of difference that manifests itself in the most extreme form. Emphatically asserting his difference, Milo confirms: 'Je n'ai plus d'amis parmi les hommes. Je n'aime pas ceux qui me ressemblent et je trouve les autres trop petits ou trop gros dans leur corps, leurs gestes et surtout leurs "opinions"' (15). Milo's only means of survival is a continued and extreme distancing of himself from other people which manifests itself in his sociopathic tendencies: overtly anti-social conduct, an inability to form meaningful relationships, amoralism and insensitivity. Just one example of his lack of sensitivity is found when he tells his wife: 'C'est peut-être aujourd'hui que je rencontrerai le grand amour de ma vie. Je t'aime mais ce n'est pas encore l'amour. Je bande tout le temps pour toi mais ce n'est toujours pas ça' (47).

Robert Hare asserts that sociopaths command attention because of the inordinate amount of crime they commit, psychologically eliciting fascination because of the cold, detached way in which they repeatedly harm and manipulate others.[8] Indeed, beneath a superficial veneer of sociability, Milo is characterised by a dearth of emotion. He describes one particular incident in which a motorcyclist draws up at the side of his car: 'J'ai sorti mon bras et l'ai poussé; il est tombé sur une table couverte d'oranges et de bananes' (*Mémoire*, 18). The brevity of his relation of the incident in itself reveals the level of importance he attaches to it and despite his apparent sense of achievement in carrying out these acts Milo completely dismisses their consequences, demonstrating an absolute lack of remorse for his actions. In response to Mireille's shock at his act, he simply replies: 'Il aurait pu se tuer, l'imbécile' (18).

This same sense of impenitence is demonstrated repeatedly in the series of murders Milo commits, for which he shows no sense of responsibility. Once again his descriptions of the acts themselves are reduced to a mere outlining of events which are portrayed without emotion. As Milo recites his list of victims and their fate, the language is abrupt, imagery is rare and instead direct and unsentimental description predominates. He remembers killing the daughter of Ismaël the Head teacher: 'J'ai vu leur fillette. Dans les cinq ans. J'ai pris un gros caillou…' (32). In similar language, he describes the murder of Ismaël, recalling simply: 'Le sang a giclé… Un bébé a crié… Je me suis enfui' (32). The violence of his acts sets Milo apart in a society against which he is constantly taking his revenge, his hatred of which is embodied in the dream to which he repeatedly returns: 'Pouvoir appuyer sur un bouton et faire disparaître cette putain d'humanité. Boum ! Un seul boum !' (16). Revenge is represented as cathartic, an outlet for Milo's anger,

---

8   Robert Hare, *Without Conscience: The Disturbing World of the Psychopaths Among Us* (New York: Guilford, 1999), 38.

offering a release from the repression he has suffered throughout his life. Theorists of rejection and exclusion have found that rejected individuals often respond by becoming hostile, angry and anti-social – precisely those behaviours likely to lead to further ostracism and exclusion.⁹

The 'Passing' Albino

The balance between the desire to belong and the simultaneous need to express individuality underlies the question of inclusion and exclusion. As the novels demonstrate, the balance between the two is a fine one. Belonging, with its inherent requirement to surrender a degree of individuality, is threatening when taken to extremes, as in the homogenisation of groups. Equally, as is the case for Sassine's protagonist Milo, if difference becomes all defining then the possibility of inclusion is negated. Inclusion, like its antithesis, manifests itself in many different ways and to varying degrees, and its importance is exposed by the extreme measures taken by those deemed too different so that they may attain a sense of belonging. The most radical of these measures, in terms of race, is the act of 'passing', undertaken by Milo on many occasions and in different forms. Throughout *Mémoire d'une peau*, Milo attempts to hide his albinism in different ways. He switches off the lights when he first sleeps with Rama so that his albinism will be forgotten: 'J'éteignis pour cacher mes premières faiblesses et pour ressembler à n'importe quel homme' (93). More controversially he attempts to 'pass' for *métis*.

'Passing' describes the way in which a member of a minority group attempts to be accepted as belonging to another race, ethnicity or gender, especially in the case of a person of mixed race being accepted as a member of the racial or ethnic majority. 'Passing' involves the adaptation or creation of a number of physical cues – like the colouring of skin, changing

9   See M.R. Leary (ed.), *Interpersonal Rejection* (New York: Oxford University Press, 2001), 3–20.

of hair style and clothing, as well as behavioural attributes, comportment and means of communication – in an attempt to temporarily cross what is termed in the US 'the color line'. Sassine's protagonist Milo describes how he is able to pass for *métis*: 'Je me teins les cheveux en noir, j'ai des crèmes pour ma peau et j'utilise même des trucs pour mes lèvres, alors au lieu de rester ce que je suis, je ressemble de loin à un métis' (146). Milo's desire to be recognised for *métis* rather than as a person with albinism represents a moderation of his extreme difference in favour of a less radical, but still problematic identity, in an attempt to be accepted. Such instances of passing are true to life and there are several references in secondary literature to attempts by people with albinism to 'pass'. Masha gives the example of urban women in Africa attempting to hide their albinism by perming and dying their hair.[10]

The act of 'passing' challenges the notion that an individual's racial identity can be discerned by sight, an idea termed by Linda Schlossberg the 'logic of visibility'.[11] The notion of the 'color-line' in the USA, and the Apartheid system in South Africa were based on such a division of groups on the basis of visible characteristics. 'Passing' calls attention to the constructed nature of race, revealing its fallacy. However, so long as races are perceived to constitute biologically distinct groups, with no opportunities for overlap, the constructed borders that distinguish one race from another remain to be 'passed' through. The consequences of such manipulation of racial boundaries are significant when considered in relation to colonial Africa, as the inability to recognise, identify and distinguish between Africans and Europeans, or between blacks and whites contrasts sharply with the colonial administrators' classification of their subjects in the colonies. In this context, the act of 'passing' has the potential to subvert by enabling the 'passer' to slip through the very boundaries that were designed to exclude him or her.

---

10   Masha, 'What kind of Black are you?', unpaginated.
11   Linda Schlossberg, 'Introduction: Rites of Passing', in Maria Carla Sanchez and Linda Schlossberg (eds), *Passing: Identity and Interpretation in Sexuality, Race and Religion* (New York: New York University Press, 2001), 1.

Despite a tendency in American literature to represent it as a life-changing and all-defining act, passing is not always permanent. In Milo's case it is brief and intermittent. He is seen to pass for both *métis* and for white in *Mémoire d'une peau*, indicating that passing functions not simply as an act of assimilation, but as a process of negotiation. Milo's negotiation of identity involves being both similar to and different from the cultural mainstream, at once visible and invisible, occupying a space of liminality. Elaine Ginsberg asserts that passing is fundamentally concerned with the creation, imposition, adoption or rejection of identities.[12] It concerns the boundaries established between identity categories and the cultural anxieties produced by the crossing of established boundaries. However, on a personal level, by passing as a member of the presumed 'norm', an individual is able to render his or her difference invisible, thus facilitating inclusion where previously he or she had been excluded.

Ginsberg argues that racial passing should be recognised as a means of allowing an individual creative subjectivity and Milo's fictive *métis* identity represents precisely such a contesting of racial, social and spatial boundaries in order that he might establish his own identity.[13] In an interview with Landry Wilfrid Miampika, Sassine describes his personal experiences of *métissage*:

> Je suis métissé. Mon père est arabe. Ma mère est africaine. Je suis même métissé religieusement. J'ai été chrétien. Je suis maintenant musulman. Mon père était chrétien, quand il est mort je suis devenu musulman à cause de ma mère. Et s'est branchée dessus la culture européenne à travers la culture française.[14]

Sassine's experiences reflect what Patrick Corcoran terms, 'the ambiguities and dualities inherent within the postcolonial perspective'.[15] Born to a Lebanese Christian father and a Guinean Muslim mother, Sassine's life

---

12   Elaine Ginsberg, *Passing and the Fictions of Identity*, 2.
13   Ibid., 11.
14   Landry-Wilfrid Miampika, 'Exil et marginalité: Entretien avec Williams Sassine.' *Africultures* (1995). <http://www.africultures.com/php/index.php?nav=article&no=665> [Accessed 14 May 2010].
15   Patrick Corcoran, *Lopes: Le Pleurer-Rire* (Glasgow: Glasgow Introductory Guides to French Literature, 2002), 7.

was divided between Guinea and a period in exile, and he combined a literary career with one in teaching. Racially *métis* figures are notable for their absence in Sassine's fictional work, but a number of characters who share Sassine's experiences of cultural and religious *métissage* populate his novels.

The concept of *métissage* has appeared in numerous discourses throughout history to refer to cultural encounters and the mixing of races. Thus, Gloria Onyeoziri notes, *métissage* is 'a term which [...] still carries significant traces of historical practices of oppression, psychological disturbances, sexual exploitation and struggles for the survival of cultural identities'.[16] In colonial Africa, mixed race individuals problematised the relationship between self and other, and the figure of the *métis* became inextricably intertwined with colonial histories of domination and exclusion. However, in the postcolonial era, the objectified figure of the *métis* emerged as a liberated and free speaking subject, and new models of *métissage* became available. *Métissage* materialised as a site of purposeful ambiguity, leading Françoise Lionnet to define it as 'the site of undecidability and indeterminacy', a position 'from which to challenge hegemonic languages'.[17] In these terms, Milo's adoption of a *métis* identity by 'passing' takes on greater significance.

A Mark of Belonging

Just as the act of 'passing' involves the disguising of distinguishing features and therefore a temporary concealment of racial markers, the novels of Destremau, Grainville and Sassine demonstrate that body marking or

---

16 Gloria Nne Onyeoziri, 'Henri Lopes and the Postcolonial Riddle of Métis Identity', *International Journal of Francophone Studies* 6.1 (2003): 43–52 (43).

17 Françoise Lionnet, *Race, Gender, Self-Portraiture* (New York: Cornell University Press, 1991), 6.

modification can also be used to emphasise allegiance to certain groups. Body modification is the deliberate, permanent or semi-permanent alteration of the body for non-medical purposes. It can range from socially acceptable body decoration such as tattooing and ear piercing, to religiously mandated alterations to the body such as circumcision. As Mike Featherstone observes, the now-acceptable use of plastic surgery to change and/or to beautify the body lies on a continuum with the more extreme acts such as subdermal implants and tongue-splitting, which are designed to assert difference.[18] In contemporary studies of the body, the dichotomy of the hidden interior and the exposed exterior is deemed central to notions of being and identity, for the exterior is associated with the social, as a means by which an individual interacts with the world.[19] Hence the importance of body modification which, in providing the opportunity to take control of the body by modifying its appearance, allows individuals to shape or to declare their identity.[20] Altering the appearance of the body also implies a sense of control over the body and its meanings; it is quite literally a means of 'constructing' identity and has been used both as a means of normalising the body considered to be abnormal or lacking and as a means of asserting and celebrating the uniqueness of an individual body in contrast to the perceived 'standard'.

Different forms of bodily marking are found in the novels of Destremau, Grainville and Sassine. References to the marking of the body by both tattooing and scarification are found in Destremau's *Nègre blanc* and Grainville's *Le Tyran éternel*. Both forms of marking the skin have long served as projects of differentiation between insiders and outsiders. Historically, the tattoo has been taken to mark off entire communities from their barbarian neighbours, to declare the criminality of a convict (whether through branding, or because he has inverted this penal practice by acquiring voluntary tattoos), and more generally to inscribe various kinds of group membership, often in opposition to a dominant culture. Despite the fact that the tattoo is visible and indelible in a physical sense, the structures of

18 See Mike Featherstone (ed.), *Body Modification* (London: Sage, 2000), 3–22.
19 Connor, *The Book of Skin*, 34.
20 Victoria L. Pitts, *In the Flesh: The Cultural Politics of Body Modification* (New York: Palgrave Macmillan, 2003), 29.

exclusion and inclusion that it appears to support are also undermined by the conceptual instability of a mark which is neither inside nor outside the skin. As Albert Parry explains, the tattoo occupies a boundary status on the skin, and this is paralleled by its cultural use as a marker of difference, an index of inclusion and exclusion.[21]

In *Le Tyran éternel*, Alpha reveals the alterations made to his body by the *guérisseur*:

> 'Regardez... un jour il m'a taillé ces dents'. En effet, les incisives étaient discrètement limées, sculptées. 'C'est un signe, comme un tatouage [...]. C'est lié aussi à ma scarification'. Alpha, en souriant, tira alors le bout de sa langue et elles virent une marque, comme un sceau minuscule, tout à la pointe de la langue. (222)

The shaping of Alpha's teeth is a mark of belonging which he deems equally as important as his scarification. Scarification is a means of permanently marking the skin by cutting, and is widely performed across Africa. Not only are the scars valued aesthetically, but they are also functional, indicating an individual's lineage. Alpha reveals that his scarification was created by the *guérisseur* as a sign of his prophetic powers and that the shaping of his teeth was to represent the rays of the sun, to serve as a link back to his mother, Mamie Reine. Paradoxically, Alpha's scarification and marking by the *guérisseur* serve not to designate him as a member of the tribe, but rather to mark him apart, as they are designed to be symbolic of his prophetic powers. Hence, the distinctiveness of his albino body is augmented by the addition of other distinguishing features.

By contrast, it is a lack of marking that troubles the young Samate. We learn that his mother Mbuya has not received the ritual tattoos of the tribe, which serve as a sign of sexual maturity:

> Comme il n'existait plus qu'un seul tatoueur rituel dans la région et qu'il était très sollicité, ses compagnes comme elle-même n'avaient pas été marquées au bas de l'abdomen et au dos des épaules, signe indiquant que les rites d'initiation avaient été menés à bien et que la future fiancée possédait les connaissances requises. (*Nègre blanc*, 89)

---

21   Albert Parry, *Tattoo: Secrets of a Strange Art* (New York: Dover Publications, 2006), 23.

The elders of the tribe overlook the marking of its young women for the practical reason that no tattooist is available. Yet, despite the apparent insignificance of Mbuya's own lack of tribal markings, the fact that Samate has not been initiated into the tribe as an infant is seen by his mother as symbolic of his non-belonging and a sign that he is to be killed. The tribe consider that circumcision, like the tattooing of the woman's body, is representative of the passage of an individual into adulthood, an altering of the appearance of the body that is symbolic of a particular identity as a boy becomes a man.

Mémoire d'une peau portrays 'passing' as an act that involves not only an altering of physical appearance, but also a change in an individual's behaviour. While for the person with albinism changing the appearance of the body often results in a loss of the defining characteristics of the condition, the assertion of particular characteristics that match the adopted identity results in the necessary relinquishing or suppressing of certain aspects of an individual's identity in order to assert others. This brings us back to the concept of 'alternative identities' mentioned earlier in this study and to the possibility of opting for a more favourable identity. Manifestations of mutually exclusive identities can be found in all four novels, but more often the sense of overlapping, complementary or parallel loci of identity is portrayed. The notion of alternative identities offers a challenge to dominant hegemonic ideologies in that the constantly changing other cannot easily be known or categorised. However, the constraints of reality on the enacting of alternative identities become evident from the texts explored here, revealing the choice between these possible identities to be inextricably associated with the acceptance of alternative social, economic and political conditions.

Destremau's Samate illustrates the switching between different identities most explicitly. He is an individual who is forced to adapt his behaviour to suit his surroundings. Caught between two worlds, with allegiances to his mother's tribe in Mozambique and to Rhodesia, the country of his adoptive father, Samate is perpetually forced to adapt. Metaphorically speaking, he must constantly change his colour to suit his surroundings and it is not insignificant that the boy has a pet chameleon. Although the whiteness of Samate's skin does not in itself change, the way in which it is interpreted and the resultant modification of his behaviour reveal the malleability of skin colour and its connotations.

The white skin that made Samate's existence in the tribe so problematic is the very same white skin that allows him privileged access to the school in his father's village:

> L'établissement est en priorité destiné aux enfants blancs, et ceux des ouvriers agricoles africains n'y sont admis qu'au compte-gouttes. Son statut de résident dans une famille connue et blanche, l'aura de son père, voire la véritable et paradoxale couleur de sa peau avaient favorisé son intégration. (*Nègre blanc*, 242)

Paradoxically, this integration comes at a cost as Samate's education exemplifies the workings of the colonial system and the process of lactification that results in '[les] transformations du sauvage inculte en un jeune homme acquérant une éducation et une culture ne déparant pas dans le milieu plutôt rustre de la société rurale' (243). This recalls Fanon's explanation of the alienation of the black child through education in *Peau noire, masques blancs* as he describes the experience of the black schoolboy who is taught at school about 'nos ancêtres, les Gaulois' and consequently comes to identify with the white man who carries truth to the savages. That is to say, an 'all-white' truth.[22] In his study of francophone sub-Saharan Africa, Patrick Manning remarks:

> In the French colonies, a commonly used text began with the words, 'our ancestors, the Gauls, were tall and blond'. The phrase, often recited by African leaders in the era of decolonization, came to symbolize the cultural imperialism of the French, and the insensitivity to African culture which this entailed.[23]

The effect of the colonial education system in Africa was profound, for the instruction of the African élite in turn influenced the social, political and economic structures of African nations to the extent that, as Gadjigo recognises: 'l'école coloniale est solidaire de la situation coloniale'.[24] Implicit in Samate's integration into the colonial education system is the boy's loss

---

22   Fanon, *Peau noire, masques blancs*, 16.
23   Patrick Manning, *Francophone Sub-Saharan Africa 1880–1995* (Cambridge: Cambridge University Press, 1995), 166.
24   Gadjigo, *Ecole blanche, Afrique noire*, 142.

of affiliation to his own culture. In the same way, the threat to Samate's identification as a black African person with albinism is manifest in his experience of the colonial education system and the process of lactification embedded within.

The Cost of Inclusion

The desire to belong and be included is evidenced in the lengths to which the protagonists of these texts go so that they might be accepted. There is a sense that Samate does ultimately attain a certain degree of belonging:

> Ainsi Samate, le petit sauvage renié de sa tribu d'origine, transposé dans un milieu pour lequel il n'était en aucune façon préparé, le petit nègre blanc fragilisé par une sensibilité physique comme sentimentale, est parvenu à s'adapter à cette nouvelle atmosphère et à y vivre raisonnablement heureux et équilibré. (*Nègre blanc*, 249)

Even the attitudes of those around him are seen to change, facilitating his integration into his adoptive father's community. The most evident change in attitude towards Samate comes from the children who had previously taunted him, but who now invite him to join in with games and share their secrets with him. Yet Samate is never to be seen simply as another person, but always as the *nègre blanc*. Despite the possibility that the boy's skin might render him more acceptable in white society, Mafavuca reminds us that Samate will never be fully accepted because '[la] peau blanche de l'enfant n'en fait pas un Européen, loin de là, et ce serait une imposture que de lui faire croire qu'il bénéficiera automatiquement en Rhodésie de cette supériorité des allogènes blancs sur les natifs noirs' (212). The strange whiteness of Samate's skin fails to elevate him to the rank of 'European' and the benefits associated with this status. Thus, the concept of 'whiteness' as a power-laden formation that privileges, secures and normalises the cultural space of the white Western subject is protected and preserved.

The novels suggest that for the person with albinism, even the smallest possibility of belonging has a cost, for it becomes apparent that belonging necessitates either a degree of conformity or a positive assertion of difference. Changes in behaviour can be seen in all four novels as the protagonists are forced to become either subservient or more radical so that they might be accepted, whether under the terms of the established 'norm' or in their extreme difference from it. Samate finds that attempts to align the disparate elements of his identity – his attachment to his mother and his simultaneous desire for the approval of his adoptive father – bring about a profound sense of discomfort:

> Il sent qu'il vit une dichotomie insupportable, une double vie dont les éléments disparates cohabitent mal en lui. L'existence dans ce cadre civilisé, ordonné, orienté vers un but, celui de le préparer à y édifier sa place au soleil, c'est-à-dire s'y intégrer définitivement sans rémission selon une logique à laquelle il n'adhère pas, il la subit sans enthousiasme ni conviction. (256)

Samate is forced to change his attitude and repress certain aspects of his personality so that he might be accepted.

In a very different way, but with the same consequences, Milo also illustrates this 'othering of the self':

> J'apprenais à devenir l'amant de poche des grandes dames, l'albinos d'occasion, très facile à plaindre, à déshabiller comme on épluche un oignon, pelure après pelure, solitude après solitude et je les regardais chercher au fond des choses. Je savais qu'au fond on se noie. (*Mémoire*, 120)

The layering described here by Milo brings to mind Connor's reference to skin colour as a layer in *The Book of Skin*. Discussing the derivation of the word 'colour', Connor notes that 'colour harbours the idea of something that both touches the skin, and is also itself, according to a curious logic of contagious replication, a kind of second skin, a layer, film or veil'.[25] Given the centrality of Milo's skin colour to his life, the peeling away of clothes can also be interpreted as a peeling away of this second skin to reveal what

---

25   Connor, *The Book of Skin*, 151.

Inclusion and Exclusion 105

lies beneath. The peeling away of layers also emerges as significant when considering Milo's construction of multiple identities, a manipulation of self identity that operates throughout *Mémoire d'une peau*.

At different times Milo is seen to present himself differently as a means of controlling the way in which others perceive him. While in the presence of his wife he often plays the role of absent, inept and downtrodden husband, but he is a loving and caring father to his children. He is ruthless in his control of his lovers, but open to manipulation by Rama. Then there is the hidden side of his personality, the voice in his head and his murderous nature that reveal a cold and calculating side to his personality. Milo is a fascinating character, portrayed by Sassine as a complex individual in a world in which he is misunderstood and even feared. While Samate is forced to emphasise or conceal different aspects of his identity at different times in order to conform to expectations, Milo uses the very malleability of identity as a means of manipulating others and constantly engineering a sense of self. His masquerading involves not only the disguising of his external appearance, but also the altering of his behaviour. Just as disguising the body provides detachment from identity, it allows for a detachment from morality and, as Chapter 5 explores, renders Milo's manipulation of identity subversive.

Mineke Schipper argues that as soon as people feel threatened, they attach great importance to their group identity.[26] However, affiliation to a group is problematised for people with albinism because, they often face rejection by others in their family or community. Equally, association with other people with albinism is difficult because many live in isolation and few, especially in rural communities, will encounter another person with the same condition in their lifetime. The development of modern communications and technologies has facilitated contact between people with the condition and in some parts of Africa it is now possible for people with albinism, who would otherwise have been isolated, to share their experiences and to seek advice from others with the same condition through support groups. However, there is equally a degree of reluctance among some

---

26   Mineke Schipper, *Imagining Insiders: Africa and the Question of Belonging* (London: Cassell, 1999), 5.

people with albinism to associate with others. As Masha notes, 'Albinos avoid each other on the bus because they don't want to draw attention to themselves. Some albinos think they are better off than others and won't be associated'.[27] In this case, certain individuals imagine that belonging to one group implicitly means exclusion from another. In the case of a group considered different or inferior, this is often so, as the individuals considered to 'belong' to a certain group risk being stigmatised by the traits considered to be typical of that group. Yet the need to belong has long been shown to be of such importance that without a sense of belonging, individuals suffer mental and physical illness. In *Mémoire d'une peau*, Milo experiences overwhelming solitude when he has finally attained a sense of belonging only for it to be taken away again. His intimate relationship with Rama and Christian is Milo's first experience of love and permits him a degree of happiness that he has not known before. His profound sense of loss at their departure is evoked in the final letter he writes to Rama:

> Chers amis. Quand je vous reverrai tout à l'heure, je vous demanderai de n'ouvrir cette lettre que dans l'avion pour des raisons de pudeur. Je vous imaginerai là-haut et moi en bas, le regard levé, levant le cœur. Si jamais vous me lisiez jusqu'au dernier mot, sachez qu'elle exprime la solitude d'un homme en plusieurs versions, de la race de ceux à qui on a arraché l'enfance et qui n'ont pas d'avenir. (156)

A reference to the multiple identities imposed on him as a person with albinism, and to the creation and adoption of identities by Milo himself, the letter conveys his extreme solitude. Milo expresses a desire for shared experience which is negated on so many levels: by the denial of access to white society, by the problematic representation of him as white when he identifies as black, by a lack of acceptance in black society and by the impossibility of associating with other people with albinism. Milo's experience reflects the reality for many people with the condition who remain isolated in rural parts of contemporary Africa.

27   Masha, 'What Kind of Black are You?'

Inclusion and Exclusion 107

The actuality of this isolation is played out in Sassine's *Wirriyamu* when Condélo admits to his dog Patience:

> Je n'ai jamais vu un albinos. Est-ce que je suis le seul albinos sur la terre? De notre petit avion, nous regarderons partout; s'il n'y en a nulle part, si je suis vraiment l'unique albinos du monde, je prierai notre maman de nous en envoyer un autre. A trois, nous nous amuserons bien! (84)

Throughout the narrative, Condélo asks this same question repeatedly, expressing his desire for shared experience, but finds that he is the only known person with albinism in the region. Although the reader is made aware of the reasons for this – the other people with albinism having been sacrificed – and despite the constant denial of the presence of others like him in the region by all the people he asks, Condélo stubbornly continues his search. He is portrayed as a lost soul without other people with whom he can identify, who dreams of a community made up of 'les albinos de toutes les couleurs et de toutes les espèces' (85). Condélo's is a utopian vision of a world where skin colours are both changeable and interchangeable, in which racial differences are erased and people judged by qualities other than their skin colour, a racial utopia of colour-blindness.

Condélo encapsulates his experience in a simple remark: 'être albinos c'est surtout se croire étranger aux autres' (104). Not only is he marked as different, but in the constant enforcement of this difference he is made to live out its consequences, his sense of non-belonging continually reinforced by a lack of recognition of the albino body by blacks and whites alike. Whereas the white sees his likeness in the albino before becoming aware of his or her black features, the black fails to recognise the 'blackness' of the albino because of the whiteness of his skin. Blankenberg discusses this problematic lack of recognition, giving an example of the momentary misrecognition of the albino by other blacks. Blankenberg refers to the moment of recognition between blacks in the West as, 'the nod of recognition' (which, she notes, may or may not occur). Rewriting this as 'the nod and the stare' she comments that:

> For the albino, the second of identification passes, is stretched out in time, as the brain absorbs the trick that the eye is playing. The totality of the image seems African – the hair, the nose, the facial structure – but the colour is incompatible. What is, is not what seems. There is no nod, only a look, and a deep, pensive scrutiny.[28]

The same moment of (mis)recognition occurs in György Sebestyén's *A Man too White*.[29] However, this time it is a moment of mis-identification of the white body on the part of the person with albinism, symbolic of his seeking his likeness in another. The protagonist recalls:

> I knew no albino except myself. Sometimes, in the street, I would see a man who was very blond and I would think, 'There's one. At last.' He would look me in the eyes for a second as he walked past and I saw that he was not an albino, merely blond. I know that look well.[30]

This desire to find his likeness in another person is momentarily realised by Destremau's protagonist Samate, but only in mis-recognition of the whiteness of the man he and his mother find lying injured in the forest:

> Samate ne se lasse pas de contempler l'homme blanc avachi à ses côtés. Moins bronzées que les bras, certaines parties de sa poitrine découverte présentent des similitudes troublantes avec sa propre peau, et le petit garçon est fasciné par la présence d'un individu possédant les mêmes caractéristiques que les siennes. Il place son bras laiteux aux côtés d'une hanche du blessé, la tourne dans un sens puis dans l'autre, émerveillé. Il a trouvé son semblable. (*Nègre blanc*, 153)

Despite the outward appearance of the man, his experience and identification as white could not be in more direct contrast with Samate's identity as a black African with albinism, something the young boy only comes to understand later. The consequent realisation that the skin colour of the other has been misrecognised is portrayed in all three texts as agonising, constituting as it does a simultaneous confirmation and reassertion of difference.

---

28   Blankenberg, 'That Rare and Random Tribe', 34.
29   György Sebestyén, *A Man too White* (Riverside, CA: Ariadne Press, 1993).
30   Ibid., 144.

Grainville's protagonist Alpha fulfils the desire for association with other people with albinism in his encounter with Salif Keita, a famous singer from Mali who is known worldwide as 'The Golden Voice of Mali'. Keita's albinism was considered a bad omen in Mali and he was alienated by his family and community. He turned to music as a means by which to use his talents and to delineate a positive identity for himself. For Alpha, the meeting with another person with the same condition is a moment of shared understanding that brings the realisation that his experience is not unique. From the outside, the two are seen and described in terms of their albinism and the whiteness that marks them both apart from the narrator, Houphouët-Boigny. However, the conversation between the two is a moment of revelation for Alpha as he recognises his own experiences in Keita's:

> Le soir, Salif Keita rencontre Alpha... Deux d'un coup! Le duo des blêmes. Salif Keita, bonnet de chanvre orné de deux cornes de gazelle, boubou blanc semé de motifs marron. Il regarde longuement le fils de Masseni. Il écoute son histoire. Tout à coup, il allonge le bras, la main. Il a une espèce de caresse bienfaisante sur la joue d'Alpha. Il parle... Salif Keita parle de son enfance. Son père et sa mère reculant effrayés devant cette engeance inexplicable. Ce fils blanchâtre qui vient de naître. Ils le rejettent, l'abandonnent aussitôt. Salif raconte son calvaire, son errance. Sa plaie. (301–2)

In the few words he speaks to Alpha, Salif confirms the commonality of albino experience, describing society's abhorrence of people with albinism who are typically persecuted and rejected. As he relates his experiences there is a sense of shared understanding between the two, 'Et l'Autre l'écoute, se reconnaît' (302). The feeling of recognition that this invokes in Alpha constitutes his first experience of sameness and his first sight of his likeness in the other person with albinism. With this recognition comes a sense of belonging and the security it affords.

However, the meeting of Alpha and Salif in Grainville's *Le Tyran éternel* is the only meeting of two people with albinism in all four novels, reflecting the lack of an albino community. For the person with albinism, often the only sense of shared experience that is possible is an association with other disabled or marginalised individuals, but as previous chapters have made clear, this can also be problematic. Hence, it is often a realisation of non-belonging that is the catalyst for the defining of albino identity. Samate confirms: 'Je *ne suis pas* un garçon comme les autres, tu le sais, et je *ne peux* espérer une vie conforme à celle des autres. Tu dois comprendre que je ne suis *ni* zimbabwéen, *ni* mozambicain, *ni* blanc, *ni* noir d'ailleurs...' (*Nègre blanc*, 264, my emphasis). Samate's awareness of the problematic ambiguity of his skin and its vulnerability to misinterpretation is revealed in his comment that he is neither Zimbabwean nor Mozambican.[31] Asserting his difference, Samate defines himself in relation to all that he 'is not'.

Samate does eventually find acceptance, but it is through the careful mediation of different aspects of his identity:

> Le jeune Tsonga a retrouvé un clan, l'élan que procure l'appartenance à un groupe. Il a créé une communauté partageant les mêmes buts, à l'image de celle au sein de laquelle évoluaient son père, sa mère et ses ancêtres. Certes, ce n'est plus un village de paillotes, une conglomération d'humains liés par la race, les croyances et les traditions. Mais ce clan n'en partage pas moins de fortes valeurs que chacun, avec ses talents reçus ou développés, contribue à défendre et à promouvoir. (285)

As a result of his creation of a music group Samate is able, to some extent, to move beyond his identification as albino. The language used posits the music group as a replacement for Samate's lost family, which it can never replace, but that nevertheless permits him a sense of belonging. At last he has found an identity that for once is not defined in terms of the standards or criteria of normality that he clearly does not meet, but that locates value and individual worth elsewhere.

In *Wirriyamu*, Condélo's dreams are replete with the need to be included, perhaps because of the impossibility of finding a sense of belonging in the community from which he has been chased. He fantasises about creating a world in which all are equal by using the sun:

> Sais-tu ce que nous en ferons ? J'ai mon plan ; si je te le montrais, tu serais fier de moi... Un jour, nous l'amènerons au-dessus du monde, tout près des têtes, et hop ! tous les cheveux seront crépus, et hop ! toutes les peaux seront noires. Moi aussi

---

31 The first part of the narrative is set in Mozambique and Rhodesia, whereas the latter part of the action, from Chapter 6 onwards, takes place in independent Zimbabwe.

Inclusion and Exclusion

je m'arrêterai sous sa douche égalisatrice, et hop ! plus d'albinos. Et lorsque j'aurai terminé, nous pourrons nous promener parmi eux, sans crainte. Est-ce qu'ils seront contents, Patience, de n'avoir plus leur albinos ? (*Wirriyamu*, 52)

Condélo's final question is pertinent, given the necessity of an other against which the 'norm' can be defined. For, as previously noted, definition of the 'normal' requires the construction of the deviant, the 'different', the 'excluded', the other, in order to define the bounds of acceptability. Condélo imagines that the 'douche égalisatrice' of the sun's rays will eliminate albinism, which is intriguing, given the damaging consequences of exposing his albino skin to it. However, his wish to appear no different from others and to be able to walk without fear is echoed in much of the literature on albinism and in many of the interviews with people with albinism that have been conducted.[32] In a world in which colour is all-defining, such a possibility can only be achieved by attempting to 'pass for normal', just as Sassine's other albino protagonist Milo passes by tinting his skin. Passing would indeed offer Condélo the potential for anonymity, but the underlying critique of the contingent nature of skin colour cannot be ignored. His later dream of a world in which there are neither Blacks, nor Whites, nor people with albinism is more utopian still. For, should skin colour and the complexities of race that are bound up in it be rendered inexistent, many of the boundaries that render albino identity so problematic would be removed.

The focus of this chapter on the construction of boundaries as a means of imposing limits and the consequent exclusion of people with albinism from society reveals a preoccupation in the work of these writers and others with where to locate the albino in relation to society. The novels portray the manner in which the figure of the albino is set apart and denied inclusion by the assertion of his difference. Whether physically excluded, ostracised or forced to 'voluntarily' distance himself from society, the fact of the person with albinism's difference is inescapable. Not only does this influence the way in which he or she is identified, but it is also seen to provoke such

---

32 See for example Archie W. Roy and Robin Spinks, *Real Lives: Personal and Photographic Perspectives on Albinism* (Glasgow: Albinism Fellowship, 2005).

extreme behaviours as 'passing' and the altering of either external appearance or the changing of mindset in order to 'fit' and attain some sense of belonging. In revealing the means and consequences of excluding people with albinism, the novels of Destremau, Grainville and Sassine interrogate the essentialism in which identity politics is grounded. At the same time they present protagonists who experiment with multiple and varied subject positions in order to cross boundaries that would otherwise exclude them, and postulate opportunities for the creation of alternative identities.

Exclusion is a word that carries many negative connotations. The concept of marginality, on the other hand, is more ambivalent: it connotes positivity and negativity, fear and fascination, repulsion and admiration. To be on the 'margins' or to inhabit the boundary itself evades the limitations demanded by notions of 'belonging' and inclusion. While, belonging implies acceptance by a group, a sense of identity and even a feeling of power. It also suggests compliance with a set of rules that render individuals acceptable within that group, but which in turn requires a series of obligations and constraints. The margin though, emerges as a new space of possibilities, a 'third space' such as that posited by Bhabha, where new subjectivities can be created and lived out. The following chapter discusses margins and liminal spaces as places of possibility and explores the potential that arises from displacing the difference of the albino to such spaces.

CHAPTER 4

Inhabiting the Margins

> Liminal space, in-between the designations of identity, becomes the process of symbolic interaction, the connective tissue that constructs the difference between upper and lower, black and white [...] the temporal movement and passage that it allows prevents identities at either end of it from settling into primordial polarities. The interstitial passage between fixed identifications opens up the possibility of a cultural hybridity that entertains difference without an assumed or imposed hierarchy.
> — HOMI BHABHA, *The Location of Culture*, 4

Characters with albinism in the novels of Destremau, Grainville and Sassine are defined by their otherness, set apart from society and placed firmly at the margins. In this sense the novels can be seen as representative of all fictional writing about albinism since, irrespective of the background of the writer, the cultural context of the work or its subject matter, writers of fiction insistently locate the figure of the albino at the margins, as a mysterious, excluded figure. However, Chevrier signals the possibilities of the margins in his study of Sassine's fictional work, suggesting that the margin is an interstitial space, 'entre l'ici et l'ailleurs, espace que l'on peut aussi qualifier, sans que la formule soit nécessairement péjorative, de "non-lieu"'.[1] Indeed, where Destremau, Grainville, and Sassine in particular, do succeed is in resisting the tendency to portray the marginality of people with albinism as purely negative. Preferring to portray the margins as a space removed from the constraints of society, these writers present the marginal spaces of their novels as, to use Bhabha's term, an 'interstitial

---

[1] Chevrier, *Le Lecteur d'Afriques*, 295.

passage', a locus of agency in which albino identity can be performed and contested.² The margin becomes a space of creativity and revolution in *Mémoire d'une peau*, *Nègre blanc*, *Wirriyamu* and *Le Tyran éternel*, in turn enabling a subversive slippage of identity and power.

Borders, Boundaries and Divisions

Grainville's description of Alpha as 'égaré, interloqué, sorti du lot, en dehors de la vie' (*Tyran*, 186) illustrates how the fundamental concept of the boundary as a dividing line is used as a means by which to define and exclude the other in terms of the politics of difference, that is to say, in accordance with the ideological legitimisation of who should and should not be included. As the previous chapter made clear, borders and boundaries have long been posited as divisions between categories, and binary order determines our understanding of the boundary. It is undeniable that boundaries provide order to experience and space, yet as this study has illustrated, the drawing of these boundaries requires that certain people and behaviours be excluded.

The boundary is used to mark the centre/margin dichotomy in all four novels explored here, and it becomes fundamental to the representation of the ambiguous position of the albino. As in much writing about people with albinism, Destremau, Grainville and Sassine depict the albino as a figure who is removed from the centre in these narratives, firmly positioned at the margins by constant reminders of his otherness. The language used to describe albinism both reflects and contributes to this marginalisation. Grainville's protagonist is described as 'le Tout Autre' (*Tyran*, 233), the translation of '*der ganz andere*' being an allusion to the albino's status as a mysterious, sacred figure. Destremau's Mbuya also refers to her child as 'un de ces humains extraordinaires' (*Nègre blanc*, 30) and Sassine's Condélo is

2   Bhabha, *The Location of Culture*, 4.

'un albinos cent pour cent' (*Wirriyamu*, 50). All three descriptions mark the albino apart from those around him by confirming his difference. A similar tendency can be found in Namba Roy's *Black Albino* in an attempt to explain the presence of the albino child in terms of the set of beliefs that render his existence so troubling. The midwife in Roy's *Black Albino* has brought hundreds of children into the world, but we learn that '[s]he had not seen an albino before, though she had heard of such a birth in her girlhood days in Africa. *Dundoes* was the name they called such children. She did not know whether it was a bad or good omen to have such a birth in the tribe' (*Black Albino*, 25).

Grainville overcomes this 'exclusion by boundaries' in the narrative layering that operates in *Le Tyran éternel*. By setting up multiple centres and margins, he draws attention to the many different levels of inclusion and exclusion at work in the society of Yamoussoukro. Houphouët-Boigny asserts his absolute control of the city: 'Ma légende est un bloc. Du marbre. Du carrare. Pas de moisi. Pas de noise' (233). However, he recognises the threat posed by his albino son, for whom he allows no space: 'Le Tout Autre n'a pu se loger dans un édifice si concerté. Cet asticot. Pas la place. Pas le moindre interstice pour ce termite blanchâtre' (233). In his use of the term *interstices*, Grainville moves beyond the designation of the boundary as a simple divide to posit the boundary as a confluence, a point at which disparate or opposing elements are fused. Because they symbolise more than simply a division between two entities, the suggestion is that interstices, or marginal spaces such as those occupied by Houphouët-Boigny's albino son, are deemed threatening to the solidity of Yamoussoukro.

Boundaries have long been described in metaphorical and symbolic terms, and been taken to refer variously to spaces 'in-between', to holes, meeting places, interfaces or sites of exchange. The notion of the margin as a hole is perhaps the most negative of these, for a hole implies a void, a space that must be filled, or more subversively perhaps, a fissure or an outlet. These descriptions have a wealth of meanings attached to them, but what is significant is that collectively they signal a movement away from the notion of the boundary as a dividing line, the same movement that is reflected in postcolonial theory in the tendency towards consideration of the boundary as an entity that can be negotiated, inhabited or broken down from within. Bhabha defines such sites as 'connective tissue that constructs the difference between upper and lower, black and white'.[3] These sites are located at the border between one condition or place and another, lodged between stable categories. The significance of this marginal space is evident in the wealth of critical attention it has received from postcolonial theorists. Following Bhabha, Pnina Werbner suggests that these 'liminal spaces [are] betwixt-and-between tropes that render authority structures ambivalent'.[4] Representing porous boundaries at which commonplaces collide and the stability of categories is subverted, the margins become the locus of ambiguity and indeterminacy, and are consequently represented as a space of agency.

The Threat of the Ambiguous

Fictional writing about albinism is replete with references to the 'in-between' status of the figure of the albino, and the narratives of Destremau, Grainville and Sassine replicate this. While Destremau's Samate is described as 'un de ces horribles individus, ni carpe ni lapin, une de ces aberrations dont la nature accouche par moments, comme dans un hoquet' (*Nègre blanc*, 29), in Grainville's *Le Tyran éternel* Houphouët-Boigny describes Alpha as 'Trop informe, trop hybride, trop avorté' (*Tyran*, 30). In their use of such language, the writers confirm that it is the indefinable nature of the albino body that renders it so troubling. The need to locate the albino body as deviant, to clearly differentiate it from the 'norm' and its consequent failure to comply, underscore its ambivalent nature and make explicit the threat it poses. This approach takes on further significance when considered in relation

---

3   Bhabha, *The Location of Culture*, 4.
4   Pnina Werbner, 'The Limits of Cultural Hybridity: On Ritual Monsters, Poetic Licence and Contested Postcolonial Purifications', *Journal of the Royal Anthropological Institute*, 184 (2001) 133–52 (141).

Inhabiting the Margins

to the anthropologist Mary Douglas's classic study, *Purity and Danger: An Analysis of Concepts of Pollution and Taboo*.[5] Douglas's recognition that the confusion of categories is frequently perceived as a form of pollution is of particular relevance to the way in which Destremau, Grainville and Sassine represent their protagonists. Douglas argues that, 'phenomena of any kind that are considered to violate the prevailing norms are usually judged dirty or polluting'.[6] Her analysis of pollution recalls colonial notions of the purity of race and culture, inherent in which was an abhorrence of racial assimilation. Consequently, the colonisers placed great emphasis on the drawing of boundaries between racial and ethnic groups to prevent their mixing. Douglas suggests that societies are likely to see individuals or objects as 'taboo' when they are anomalous, when they do not fit neatly into a society's classification of the world. She argues that entities which exist at the borders of society or on the boundaries between categories are perceived as possessing both power and danger, suggesting that for some purposes the power may be stressed, and for others the danger.

Douglas's observations have clear relevance to a reading of the novels examined here, in which the notion of the body of the albino as polluting is closely linked to the disgust felt towards it. This sense of disgust is epitomised in Sassine's *Wirriyamu* in the black soldier's description of Condélo's skin:

> Tout était si froid au toucher! Ça me rappelle les petits lézards tout blancs des murs, je crois qu'on les appelle geckos. Oui, c'est ça, il m'a donné l'impression d'un coup d'être un gecko ; et c'est cette impression qui vous reste collée à la peau comme une saleté dès que vous le touchez. (90)

Sassine's use of the word 'saleté' in relation to the albino body brings to mind the threat of contamination or pollution associated with it. Condélo's skin is intolerable to the soldier and the revulsion felt towards it is closely allied with its enigmatic colour and the inability of the soldier to label the

---

5 Mary Douglas, *Purity and Danger: An Analysis of Concepts of Pollution and Taboo* (London: Routledge, 1966).
6 Ibid., 114.

boy as either black or white. Grainville's Houphouët-Boigny attributes this ambiguity to people with albinism in general: 'Des Nègres blancs, des Nègres roses, des Nègres neigeux. Des monstres, si tu veux. Incomplets, inachevés, sans derme définitif' (*Tyran*, 26). The loss of definition between the body and the outside world – being without a skin – is signalled as troubling, for as I remark in Chapter 1, the loss of bodily boundaries defies the need to contain and to control.

Douglas conceptualises the threat to order in terms of the body as a symbol of society, arguing that social pollution is always a sign of the existence of an order: what does not fit into the confines of a certain social order is cast out as 'unclean'. She argues that to be able to understand body pollution, 'we should try to argue back from the known dangers of the society to the known selection of bodily themes and try to recognise what appositeness is there'.[7] Cultural symbolism, Douglas argues, organises conventional reality into tidy categories, and so departures from these are regarded in many cultures as dangerous. The disabled fall into the category of the contaminated for this reason: they are anomalies. In his study on disability, Robert Murphy describes how some disabilities disturb the able-bodied more than others:

> There is a hierarchy of devaluation that varies with severity and type of disability. At the bottom of the scale are persons with facial disfigurement or marked body distortion; wheelchairs are somewhere in the middle. The main criterion seems to be based on the extent to which one differs from the standard human form.[8]

As Murphy notes, one can add to Douglas's theory Lévi-Strauss's idea that the greatest of all binary distinctions in human thought is the separation of nature and culture. Within the framework of this dualism, the physical impairment of albinism becomes not only an infringement by nature, but also an intrusion that undercuts an individual's status as a bearer of culture. Murphy argues that this relationship between nature and culture is what renders disability of any kind so different from other kinds

---

7   Ibid., 121.
8   Robert Murphy, 'Encounters', 154.

of deviance, 'for it is not merely a departure from the moral code, but a distortion of conventional classification and understanding.'[9] Equally, the figure of the albino is a symbol of otherness in fictional representation, a multiply marginalised figure that complicates and unbalances. However, this very unbalancing challenges normality and its stereotypes to search for the crucial point at which the human being can be accepted as being 'fully human'. As I shall discuss later, this demands a reconsideration of the limits of acceptability, and in so doing, requires new parameters for our understanding of the world.

While the figure of the albino inhabits a liminal space on the boundaries of society, physical acceptability and race, the ambiguous nature of his body permits a certain freedom. The portrayal of Sassine's Milo illustrates this most clearly as he passes for *métis* and manipulates his identity throughout *Mémoire d'une peau*. Although 'passing' is usually a movement across colour boundaries from black to white, Milo's acts of passing are a move in the opposite direction, towards blackness, towards his origins and towards the racial identification of his parents. In his act of passing, Milo manipulates the ambiguity associated with the albino body; a body which is 'slippery', to use Douglas's term.[10] That is to say, it is indefinable, elusive and potentially problematic. The ambiguity embodied in the figure of the albino disturbs notions of identity and order, and signals a failure to respect borders and the rules by which they are defined.

The albino body reveals the very threat of the indefinable or the marginal to be bound up in the potential loss of distinction between self and other, a notion which is central to Kristeva's theory of the abject.[11] For Kristeva, the abject refers to the human reaction to a threatened breakdown in meaning caused by the loss of the distinction between subject and object or between self and other.[12] The primary example used by Kristeva to demonstrate what causes such a reaction is that of the corpse, as

---

9   Idem.
10 Douglas, *Purity and Danger*, 124.
11 Julia Kristeva, *Pouvoirs de l'horreur: essai sur l'abjection* (Paris: Broché, 1980).
12 Ibid., 65.

it traumatically reminds us of our own materiality.[13] The reference to the corpse is significant here, given the close and often-explicit association made between the albino body and the cadaver. In Sassine's *Wirriyamu*, Condélo is described as ressembling the dead and his skin is compared to a shroud. Grainville's Alpha is portrayed in similar terms as 'un cadavre en marche' (*Tyran*, 125).

The potential loss of distinction between self and other, subject and object, explains why the albino body is deemed to be so troublesome, for it does not distance the subject from that which threatens it, but instead acknowledges it to be in perpetual danger. For the villagers of Namba Roy's *Black Albino*, the distinction between the black albino and the white coloniser is blurred to such an extent that the people see them as one and the same:

> The people of the hills had learned to look upon a white face with fear and hate. It was their nightmare – white faces, associated with slave pens, beatings, tortures, and death – and now converted into another sign of ill omen.[14]

The danger associated with the white coloniser is transposed onto the white body of the albino, which is considered to be equally threatening, albeit in a different way. Where the whiteness of albinism is feared for its incomprehensibility, the whiteness of the coloniser brings with it associations of pain and death.

Thus the novels of Destremau, Grainville, Sassine and Roy demonstrate the possibilities inherent in the ambiguity associated with the body of the albino, particularly on the level of individual identity. In Bhabha's view, the spaces in between subject positions offer the possibility of disrupting cultural structures and practices. For, as he suggests, the existence of liminal space and the movement it permits prevents identities at either end of it from 'settling into primordial polarities'.[15] Therefore, rather than emphasising the opposition between binaries such as Africa and the West,

13 Idem.
14 Roy, *Black Albino*, 90.
15 Bhabha, *The Location of Culture*, 4.

Inhabiting the Margins

coloniser and colonised, man and woman, and black and white, Bhabha proposes that we might more profitably focus on the margins as the sites where identities are performed and contested. Ascribing the term 'hybrid' to this interstitial space, Bhabha asserts his notion of 'a cultural hybridity that entertains difference without an assumed or imposed hierarchy'.[16] In contrast to clear-cut binary oppositions, hybridity offers an unstable and ambivalent alternative because, in recognising the in-between, it permits a move beyond dualism and binary thinking that results in the transcending of binary categories and all that their presence implies.

Bhabha's notion of hybridity is a radical inversion of the negativity that was historically associated with the concept, for, positioned within or beside theories of human origin, the hybrid appears as a marker of inadequacy, contamination or regression. In colonial discourse imbued in nineteenth-century eugenicist and scientific-racist thought, 'hybrid' is a term of abuse for those who are products of miscegenation. In terms of Bhabha's theory of hybridity, *Wirriyamu*, *Mémoire d'une peau*, *Le Tyran éternel* and *Nègre blanc* highlight the potential of the figure of the albino which results from the threat his presence poses to established categories from within and without. Having elected to withdraw from a society that does not accept him, to live in the forest, Grainville's Alpha is firmly positioned on the geographical bounds of society, but is able to gain influence from this marginal space and thus the wilderness he inhabits becomes a space of resistance and agency. His eventual coming to power represents both a threat from the outside as he is refused acceptance in Yamoussoukro, but also from the inside when it emerges that he is the son of the despotic ruler Houphouët-Boigny. Alpha is described as 'l'envers étrange d'Houphouët-Boigny. Comme son double surnaturel et tabou' (*Tyran*, 231). Alpha's existence on the margins of Yamoussoukro translates into a position of agency that Sylvanus realises will ultimately permit him to challenge Houphouët Boigny's tyrannical rule.

16 Idem.

Geographical Margins

Destremau, Grainville and Sassine's choice of a marginal geographical space as the locus of the action in their novels is significant. The most important events of *Wirriyamu, Le Tyran éternel* and *Nègre blanc* take place in the forest, a space beyond the limits of 'civilisation'. *Mémoire d'une peau* is an exception, as Milo remains in the city, and marginal spaces do not take a geographical form in the novel. Not only does the forest offer the albino protagonists protection from the sun that is so damaging to their skin, but it also offers a certain freedom from physical and psychological bullying, and liberates him from cultural belief systems that inform and advocate such behaviour. It is interesting that all three writers choose the forest as the marginal space of their novels, for in traditional belief in parts of Africa, the forest is considered to be a place inhabited by *revenants*, those individuals who have not made the move from the real world to the spirit world upon their death. It is significant that Destremau, Grainville and Sassine should all choose to locate their protagonists within this space, reinforcing the enduring association of this figure with the spirit world.

The distinction between the wilderness and civilisation is a key opposition in these novels, for the wilderness connotes exactly that which civilisation is not. In Sassine's *Wirriyamu*, the cool, fresh air of the forest is set up in opposition to the stagnant, hopeless situation in the village, which is echoed in the attitude of its few remaining inhabitants:

> Prostré sur une chaise, une lueur de lassitude dans les yeux, le patron de 'La Calebasse d'or' regardait tomber la pluie. Sa petite femme, assise en face, poussait d'affreux soupirs d'énervement. (24)

The forest is a place of refuge for the protagonist Condélo and for the short time he spends in the forest, it is a place of relative freedom after the bullying and teasing he has faced in the village:

> Son chien marchait devant, à petits pas précipités, la tête au ras du chemin qui se tortillait parmi les herbes. L'albinos le suivait du même pas, reniflant avec bonheur le vent chargé de fraîcheur. Il s'arreta près d'une branche, tendit l'oreille et repartit rassuré, encore plus heureux. (83)

Inhabiting the Margins 123

Destremau and Grainville represent the forest in a similar way, as a wild, 'uncivilised' space, set up in direct contrast with the constructed, controlled and controlling spaces of the city, tribe, family and colony. Destremau's Mbuya sums up this dichotomy in her reflection on life in the forest, which she constrasts with the years she has spent living in her native village. Whereas the village is defined by customs and laws, in the forest she has the freedom to decide how she will spend her day, the only constraint being that she must ensure her survival and that of her son.

The contrast between civilisation and wilderness is also set up in Grainville's *Le Tyran éternel*. Houphouët-Boigny describes the city of Yamoussoukro that he has shaped around his own intimate designs:

> Les quatre lacs qui bordent deux à deux le boulevard central: Mamie Adjoua. Ce grand fleuve médian et macadamisé porte le nom de ma sœur défunte, de ma grande chérie morte. La cité dans son essence même n'est que l'union de nos deux corps jumelés. Au nord-ouest où nous sommes: le Palais du Président, la Basilique du Président. Un peu plus au sud, la mosquée au centre du quartier populaire, les gares, le marché grouillant. A l'est, les grandes écoles [...] Tout au sud, la Maison du Parti, l'Hotel Président, la Fondation Président. Façades de marbre et grandes esplanades d'accès. (15)

However, Sylvannus describes how the sprawl of the city stops suddenly as its roads come to an abrupt end when they meet the forest. Until Houphouët-Boigny's dream of motorway links between Yamoussoukro and the other capital cities of Africa is realised, the boundary between the city and the forest will remain clearly marked.

The very different language used to describe the two environments also signals the contrast between the two. On their first visit to the forest, Joan and July, the teenage nieces of Cécil, are at once excited and afraid, unsure as to how they should behave in their new surroundings. The forest is described as an environment that stimulates the girls' senses:

> Le soleil s'était légèrement décalé et le surplomb rocheux répandait sur leurs corps une nappe d'ombre. Elles entendaient tout. Leur écoute atteignait à une intensité prodigieuse... les moindres rumeurs, les coulées de vent, l'attaque soudaine d'un gloussement, d'une criaillerie d'oiseau, les répits, les secrets mugissements. L'âme de la forêt les enveloppait, les pressait. (167)

Grainville's portrayal of the forest as a place closely associated with sensual experience, authenticity and origins brings to mind the Western image of Africa as 'the cradle of mankind'. However, it also recalls the propensity of white colonisers to associate black Africans with the wilderness and savagery, implicit in which is the drawing of an association between whites and civilisation. Destremau, Grainville and Sassine all play with this opposition in their novels, positing the forest as a space of agency, beyond the bounds of civilisation and all that this implies.

The divide between the wilderness and civilisation that is set up in each of the novels, and particularly Grainville's *Le Tyran éternel*, recalls Fanon's 'monde coupé en deux', where a dividing line separates the clean and prosperous areas of the colonisers from the poverty and dirt of the *quartier indigène*.[17] Fanon describes the colony as a world of two irreconcilable spaces:

> La zone habitée par les colonisés n'est pas complémentaire de la zone habitée par les colons. Ces deux zones s'opposent, mais non au service d'une unité supérieure. Elles obéissent au principe d'exclusion réciproque: il n'y a pas de conciliation possible.[18]

The conflict between civilisation and wilderness is also set up in this way in the novels. However, the narratives demonstrate that the albino is able to exploit his ambiguous status to move into and out of these spaces in a crossing of boundaries that becomes more significant when the power relations associated with each of these places is taken into consideration.

Place is often perceived to be a passive space within which events occur, but the references to specific places in the novels remind us that the characters live in a tangible world which is shaped by the buildings, objects and other people that surround them. The relationships of the protagonists with these places are sometimes transient and meaningless beyond the moment in which they are experienced, as demonstrated by Condélo's experience of the forest:

---

17 Fanon, *Les Damnés de la terre*, 68–9.
18 Idem.

Inhabiting the Margins

> L'albinos cassa une branche; avant de s'en servir comme canne, il s'adressa à l'arbre: 'Pardonne-moi; j'ai besoin de quelque chose pour m'aider à monter…' Patience émit de petits grognements d'impatience; alors Condélo le rejoignit et ensemble, péniblement, ils gravirent les pentes de l'énorme montagne. (*Wirriyamu*, 85)

Although Condélo and Patience must keep moving in an effort to evade the Portuguese soldiers pursuing them, Condélo still engages with the environment through which he travels. More often though, relationships with place in the narratives are lasting and intimate, as is Samate's life-long relationship with his native village, despite his early removal from it.

Surprisingly, given his generally negative attitude, Milo too describes his attachment to the town in which he lives, replete as it is with its frustrations:

> C'était le bouchon habituel, les bonjours par les portières et autres cris de reconnaissance, les bruits de pots d'échappement crevés que rendait encore plus insupportables la première chaleur humide matinale. Le nouveau régime promettait d'agrandir les routes, de construire de nouveaux axes, et peut-être même des ponts pour contourner les difficultés. Mais il fallait commencer d'abord par casser. J'avais peur qu'on ne casse tout, bêtement, comme les anciens dirigeants. J'aime ma ville comme toutes celles sorties du passé avec des blessures. (*Mémoire*, 18)

Places are given meaning and status in each of the novels and consequently contribute to the shaping of the protagonists' sense of self. As the above quotation from Sassine's *Mémoire d'une peau* demonstrates, places also generate a range of emotions, which range in the narratives from those of pleasure and belonging, to those of exclusion and fear.

Environmental and social psychologists have long been interested in 'place identity'.[19] The concept deals with the interaction between questions of identity and how the local environment, including geographical location, influences an individual's life. At the heart of this notion of place is the need for a sense of belonging and some theorists go so far as to argue that belonging-ness is not only one aspect of place identity, but a necessary

---

19   Michael Keith, *Place and Identity* (London: Routledge, 1993).

basis for it.[20] Place theorists view individuals as imaginative 'users' of their environments, agents who are able to appropriate physical spaces in order to create a space of being. Indeed, the novels demonstrate the different ways in which individuals shape the places in which they live. Destremau's Mbuya creates a home for herself and Samate in the forest: 'Il lui faut moins de deux semaines pour adopter ce coin de savane, le considérer comme sa propriété, un lieu hospitalier ou il fera, à coup sûr, bon vivre. Elle y est chez elle' (*Nègre blanc*, 103). Grainville's Alpha also establishes a temporary home for himself in a cave, hidden away in the forest, which Joan and July discover in their search for him:

> Une fissure ouvre la pierre, une sorte de cheminée. [...] C'est le silence. Et puis, là, devant elles, à leurs pieds, dans une tache de lumière: l'amas des cendres et le bois en attente, des restes de boisson. Plus loin, une natte, un plaid, un tas de guenilles, des ustensiles de pêche, un piolet, des fruits en vrac. C'est une cache, un repaire. (*Tyran*, 114)

Thus the novels demonstrate the investment of the protagonists in certain places, tracing the claiming and consequent transformation of these places into a space of refuge, and the resulting sense of belonging.

It becomes clear that a sense of place is essential to an individual's sense of identity, but at the same time the novels reveal some places to be saturated with relations of domination and thus closely linked to an individual's position in, or on the margins of, society. Samate, Alpha and Condélo all experience physical dislocation. Whether their removal from society functions as a confirmation of marginality as in the case of Condélo, or as a means of confirming security as for Samate and Alpha, it becomes apparent that the displacement they each experience has a fundamental impact on their development as individuals.

The process of displacement is particularly bound up with the formation of identity for the protagonist of Destremau's *Nègre blanc*, which portrays the young Samate's removal from his native village and his tribe,

---

20 K.M. Korpela, 'Place-Identity as a Product of Environmental Self-Regulation', *Journal of Environmental Psychology*, 9 (1989), 241–56 (246).

Inhabiting the Margins

and his double displacement, firstly to the forest and subsequently to Rhodesia, the country of his adoptive father. The crossing from civilisation to wilderness is represented in Destremau's *Nègre blanc* as a life-changing experience for both Samate and his mother Mbuya. Fearing for her son's life, Mbuya severs her links and those of her child with family, tribe and community, believing that as a consequence, although she and her son will be safe, they will be destined to live in isolation in the forest. For Samate's mother, the departure from the village to the savannah is traumatic and the consequences are profound:

> Le franchissement de son Rubicon personnel fait d'elle une non-personne, une morte vivante portant à son côté un nègre blanc sauvé d'une mort dégradante, mais désormais voué à une existence pleine de périls insoupçonnés. (72)

For Mbuya, the crossing of the threshold is a distressing departure from all that she knows and after her initial bravado she comes to realise the implications of her act: 'Que va-t-elle faire maintenant? Appuyant la tête contre le tronc solide et rassurant, à demi étendue, la jeune femme est incapable d'imaginer son avenir' (76). Mbuya's movement beyond the bounds of civilisation into the savannah serves as confirmation that such liminal spaces are the dwelling place of those who no longer 'belong'. This idea is particularly pertinent when considered in relation to Young's commentary on civilisation:

> [T]o be civilised meant to be a citizen of the city (preferably walled), as opposed to the savage (wild man) outside or the more distant barbarian roaming in the lands beyond. It thus operated within the terms of the later ideological polarity of the country and the city, for the inhabitants of the city contrasted themselves to the savages outside.[21]

Young emphasises the need to construct and maintain the polarity of civilised and savage, wilderness and civilisation. This antithesis takes on further meaning in terms of Whatmore's depiction of the wilderness as '[A] place without *us*, populated by creatures (including, surreptitiously, a variety of

---

21   Young, *Colonial Desire*, 31.

human 'kinds') at once monstrous and wonderful, whose very strangeness gives shape to whatever *we* are claimed to be'.²² Whatmore's description recalls the need to designate a clearly defined other; the same need that is satisfied by the Freak Show. Just as the bodies of people with albinism displayed in the Freak Show confirm the normality of the onlooker, the creatures deemed to exist in the wilderness affirm the necessity of securing the boundaries of civilisation to protect the privileged within.

As a young boy Samate is particularly at home in the savannah. He revels in a close contact with his surroundings and is described as 'belonging' to the environment in which he spends his childhood: 'Sa longue pratique, sa vie entièrement immergée dans la forêt et la brousse expliquent qu'il les respire et que son cœur batte à leur unisson. Il leur appartient. C'est son unique univers' (*Nègre blanc*, 215). Yet Samate's intimate communion with the forest troubles his mother Mbuya, who fears that her child will be consumed by the very environment that has shaped him. Watching her son play in the water, she remembers an infant sacrifice that she attended as a young girl. She recalls having witnessed a baby with albinism being propelled into the water by the *sorcier-mage*, and wonders if her son is destined for the same fate:

> Quand il n'aide pas sa mère aux travaux ménagers ou agricoles, Samate vit dans l'eau, et Mbuya ne peut s'empêcher d'établir des rapprochements terrifiants: la destinée de ce nègre blanc, fils expulsé de ses entrailles, était-elle vraiment d'échapper à une déstinée marquée par l'eau ? [...] Lui, Samate, ou tous les albinos sont-ils irrémédiablement liés à l'eau, morts ou vivants, et la malédiction qui repose sur leur tête ne s'accomplira-t-elle pas un jour ou l'autre quoi qu'on fasse ? (122)

Mbuya fears that the 'exigeants hôtes' (40) that inhabit the river will reclaim her son. The river operates in *Nègre blanc* as a boundary between the spiritual world and the real world. This is particularly significant, for the threshold between the two is often perceived to be the dwelling place of spirits, ghosts and the souls of the dead. The water spirit Mami Wata,

---

22 Sarah Whatmore, *Hybrid Geographies: Natures, Cultures, Spaces* (London: Sage, 2002), 12.

Inhabiting the Margins

who is believed to be capable of bestowing blessings or inflicting mental and physical pain on those who meet her near the rivers or streams where she dwells, is just one example. In some African folk tales water, like the forest, is considered to comprise another world that is deemed to be at once a constituent part of, yet removed from, the 'real world'. Mbuya's fears that her son will return to the water are founded on the notion that people with albinism and other marginal beings belong in this intermediary space, returning to the notion that the in-between is problematic.

Samate's early displacement means that he has little with which to compare his life in the savannah, but he continues to hold a loyalty towards his native village and its people. It is not until his adulthood that he comes to understand his mother's motives for removing him from the village. Whereas Samate is portrayed as being at home in the savannah and then the forest, the white Mafavuca finds the terrain difficult to cross:

> Il avait largement sous-estimé la difficulté du terrain qui, le long de la frontière entre le Mozambique et la Rhodésie, prenait l'aspect de montagnes élevées et couvertes d'une végétation de type équatorial, dense et pratiquement infranchissable. D'en haut, vu d'un hublot d'avion ou de la porte d'un hélicoptère, le sol ne révèle pas toujours les détails de sa réalité. (223–34)

Mafavuca's failure to fully comprehend the environment in which he finds himself echoes the general tendency of colonial administrators and policy makers to view Africa from afar. His mis-reading and mis-interpretation of the African landscape is symbolic of the failure on the part of the colonisers to recognise the complexity of the cultures and the peoples they colonised. Further reinforcing this, Mafavuca's inability to deal with the terrain is set up in direct contrast to the ease with which the young Samate copes with the environment. Thus a new insider/outsider dichotomy is established that affirms Samate's identity as 'un enfant des bois' (215), an assertion of his belonging to the forest that simultaneously highlights the trespassing of the outsider Mafavuca within it. This contrasts with the situation in the colonial world in which Samate will soon find himself, where the superiority of the white over the black is enforced at every level, and where Samate will be the outsider.

The forest becomes more than a space of freedom for the young Samate. It is also a place in which he will attain his independence and make the transition from childhood into adolescence. After the death of his mother, Samate crosses the forest with his adoptive father Mafavuca. Destremau describes the journey as a reversal of that from the village into the savannah as Mafavuca and Samate travel through the wilderness towards civilisation and all that it entails:

> Cette longue marche est implicitement reconnue comme le franchissement d'un sas, le temps d'écoulement qu'il faut au fleuve des souvenirs pour s'adapter petit à petit aux nouvelles et implacables réalités de la vie et à l'inconnu qui y préside. (*Nègre blanc*, 216)

Although the journey is a time of mourning on the part of Samate after the death of his mother and a time in which he grieves for what has been left behind, it is also a period during which Mafavuca attempts to describe to Samate the world beyond the border, gradually familiarising him with the way of life in the 'civilised world':

> Comme il manque du minimum de notions de base, il est nécessaire pour le Blanc de remonter très en arrière, et parfois de faire appel à l'histoire de l'humanité pour expliquer un fait banal, voire naturel pour lui. [...] Mafavuca déploie des trésors d'ingéniosité l'évolution des habitudes humaines, les bonds énormes accomplis par ce qu'on appelle la civilisation et qu'on oppose à l'état sauvage. (*Nègre blanc*, 217)

Here Destremau draws out the binary of civilised and savage in Mafavuca's struggle to articulate to the young boy a world that he cannot understand because he lacks the necessary points of reference, and at the same time highlights the set of assumptions that underlie the binary opposition of civilised and savage.

As Mafavuca and Samate approach the edge of the savannah, the signs of the outside world become more evident and it becomes clear that lines have not only been drawn on minds and maps by the colonisers, but that artificial physical boundaries have been created in order to separate countries:

Inhabiting the Margins 131

> Progressivement, les indices de la proximité immédiate du but viennent s'accumuler et étayer leur certitude: des feux de forêts se multiplient comme si on avait l'intention de créer une zone de protection le long de la ligne artificielle séparant les deux pays. (225)

The description of the border as 'artificielle' in this quotation is evidently a commentary on the drawing of boundaries by colonial administrators as Africa was parcelled up. The 1884–1885 Berlin Conference is one of the clearest examples of the assumptions and preconceptions of this era, and its effects on Africa can still be seen today, for the arbitrary boundaries that were imposed both divided ethnic groups and brought enemies under the same government. The maps drawn by colonial administrators came to be viewed as external impositions and despite claims that such colonial 'mapping' ultimately created national identities among the multiple ethnic groups which found themselves within colonial boundaries, it is clear from the ongoing conflict throughout the African continent that colonial maps have not laid a stable basis for nationhood in Africa.

Not only is Samate's journey with Mafavuca a physical traversing of the forest towards civilisation, but it is also a journey into adulthood. He explains:

> Moi, jai été exclu de ma tribu par la fuite de ma mère pour me sauver la vie, et personne ne peut m'adouber, me délivrer ce brevet d'honorabilité. Pas de régulo ou de feiticeiro qui me présente aux autres gens du village comme un adulte nouvellement entré dans la communauté. (230)

In Samate's village, the rite of passage constitutes the transition from childhood to adulthood, marking the changed status of an individual, with the concomitant shifts in roles, responsibilities, control, and power. The ceremonial passage into adulthood marks the identity of an individual within the community and defines him in relation to both his extended family and to his lineage. It is also a process of identifying those who are permitted to belong to the group and those who are to remain without, and so it is not insignificant that Destremau's young protagonist has not been allowed the opportunity to participate in the rite of passage. Although Samate is ignorant of this, and seems to have little idea as to what exactly constitutes this tribal rite of passage, he is aware of the importance placed on the initiation and keen to confirm his manhood. He explains to Mafavuca his desire to fulfil these, commenting: '[u]n albinos non initié accumule les difficultés, n'est-ce pas?' (232). His remark anticipates the manifold difficulties he is to encounter in the outside world, but as a consequence of his albinism and not purely because of his lack of initiation.

Since Samate cannot exactly replicate the tribal rites of the village, the expedition through the forest becomes a substitute rite of passage. Samate's journey is described in terms of a loss of innocence and an initiation into the realities of the adult world: 'Ce grand parcours se rapprocherait d'une initiation rituelle due à un changement de statut du garçon, qui, devenu adolescent, bascule dans le monde cruel et exigeant des adultes' (216). Wangarĩ Nyatetũ-Waigwa describes such a passage from childhood into adulthood as the traversing of a state of liminality.[23] Nyatetũ-Waigwa draws on Victor Turner and Arnold Van Gennep's formulation of the rite of passage whereby individuals move from one status to another. For Victor Turner and Arnold Van Gennep, the process is characterised by three basic stages: separation from a previous position in life (preliminal); a period of transition or a liminal space in between both categories (liminal); and finally, incorporation to a newly conferred status (postliminal).[24] This process is closely depicted in the narrative structure of *Nègre blanc* and can be traced through the chapter headings: Le village, La savane, Mafavuca, La civilisation.

The preliminal stage separation from a previous position in life – and from a previous way of life – occurs early in Samate's childhood when his mother Mbuya decides that it is too dangerous for her son to stay within the tribe. She and Samate leave behind not only their family, tribe and village, but also the memories attached to them. Mbuya's regret is summed up in a few words: 'Les lieux appellent tous de merveilleux et impalpables souvenirs, parés des meilleures couleurs, des plus tendres invocations, et de riche signification pour celle qui sait qu'elle va les quitter pour toujours' (67).

---

23 Wangarĩ Nyatetũ-Waigwa, *The Liminal Novel: Studies in the Francophone-African Novel as Bildungsroman* (New York: Peter Lang, 1996), 94–102.
24 Victor Turner, *The Ritual Process* (New York: Aldine de Gruyter, 1969) and Arnold Van Gennep, *The Rites of Passage* (Chicago: University of Chicago Press, 1960).

Inhabiting the Margins

However, once they have broken away from all that is known, Mbuya and her son move to the liminal space of the savannah where bounded, constructed space comes to an end, giving way to a more abstract liminal space in which they are free of the confines of society and its prejudices. It is in the savannah that the young Samate meets Mafavuca, who will play a central role in his adult life.

Referring to Turner and Van Gennep's notion of the middle phase of the rite of passage, Nyatetū-Waigwa notes that the liminal phase is not purely a ritual passage, but also a physical one.[25] Certainly, Samate's ritual passage is celebrated not only in the physical movement of his journey from the wilderness to civilisation, but in a cultural initiation that is described as a move from savagery to the 'civilised world: 'Il commence sa vie d'homme civilisé' (240). It is the liminal phase of this passage that invites attention because of its problematic status as an 'in-between' space, and it is this stage of development that is the focus of Destremau's novel since it is essential to Samate's negotiation of identity. Nyatetū-Waigwa suggests that 'in-between', marginal or liminal space is particularly ambiguous and problematic as it is associated with anonymity and a temporary loss of status.[26] This moment of uncertainty experienced by Samate as he seeks to come to terms with his changing status is a decisive one. Samate's rite of passage is symbolic of his coming of age, but it is also a conscious attempt to construct and to confirm his identity, reinforcing his links to the tribe.

Multiple Centres, Multiple Margins

The constant movement of marginal subjects between different categories gives rise to an identity defined in terms of multiple subject positions and emerges as a direct challenge to the formulation of subjectivity as unitary

---

25 Nyatetū-Waigwa, *The Liminal Novel*, 93–4.
26 Ibid., 94.

and singular. Postcolonial critiques of unitary models of subjectivity reveal that all such models are based on binary thinking. Rejecting binary models, Hall, Bhabha and Spivak prefer to describe both subjectivity and experience as decentred and pluralistic. The hybrid subjectivity of the albino permits such a celebration of difference, a circumvention of the politics of polarity and of binary oppositions. At the same time, the margins emerge as the location of the decentred experience lived by people with albinism in much of sub-Saharan Africa and emerge as a challenge to notions of the centre as the sole locus of power.

This challenge to the centre emerges and is articulated in several different ways throughout the novels. Most obviously, as the first chapter of this study discussed in some detail, the albino body may be considered to be racially inadequate in relation to both blackness and whiteness, but the constructed nature of racial difference is revealed in the albino body's very exclusion from these categories which fail to account for the chromatic ambivalence resulting from albinism. Consequently, the albino body threatens to disrupt and to undermine the hierarchy of colour from within. Not only is the albino body deemed racially inadequate, but it is often considered physically incomplete, inadequate, or lacking, and is consequently defined as 'monstrous'. Yet, as Shildrick reminds us, the presence of the 'monstrous' serves as a constant reminder of the permeability of the boundaries that guarantee the normatively embodied self.[27] Ironically then, it is the authors' very insistence on the series of binaries that define the otherness of the albino that frequently draws attention to the instability of the categories that define the 'normal' individual. By marking the difference of the figure of the albino in their fictional work, the writers invite reflection on what exactly constitutes normality, for marginality is a condition necessarily constructed in relation to a privileged centre.

The centre/margin dichotomy operates on many different levels for each of the protagonists. As Destremau's *Nègre blanc* illustrates in particular, the 'centre' is not only an imperial centre that marginalises the albino as a Black other. It can also be an African centre because, whether his whiteness is feared or celebrated, the person with albinism is often cast out to the margins

---

27   Shildrick, *Embodying the Monster*, 5.

of African society. Destremau's Samate is forced to abandon his village, for his mother knows that he will be destined for sacrifice if he stays. Marginalised too in terms of deviance from the acceptable bodily norm, the person with albinism is stigmatised for his difference. In many parts of the world, albinism is not considered to constitute an 'illness' as it is not considered a progressive condition. However, there is ongoing discussion as to whether or not albinism constitutes a disability; an ambiguity that creates a problem in the language used to talk about albinism and that makes it difficult for people with albinism to identify themselves as a group. Despite the potential offered by the multiple identity positions open to people with albinism, the fact that these alternate 'centres' exist also emerges as problematic. The predominance of this idea in Sassine's work in particular suggests that it is fundamental to the albino individual's search for identity.

All three writers present the experience of marginality specific to their albino protagonists as one that can be intensely positive and profoundly negative. Chevrier argues that the concept of marginality is fundamental to an understanding of Sassine's fictional work:

> L'une des premières originalités des romans de Williams Sassine nous paraît en effet se situer dans l'attention qu'il apporte au monde des exclus, des rebelles et des marginaux de la nouvelle société africaine, une société en forme de goulag, à l'évidence placée sous le signe du malheur, de la violence et de l'oppression.[28]

In Sassine's *Wirriyamu*, Condélo is trapped in his marginality, experiencing conflicting loyalties and defined by his difference. Rather than deconstructing the typecasting of the albino as passive victim, as he does in *Mémoire d'une peau*, Sassine here presents Condélo as a scapegoat and *Wirriyamu* is, at best, the narrative of a victim. The incessant objectification of Condélo's body in repeated references to the ancestral practice of blood-letting and the value attached to his corpse define him as a tragic sacrificial victim. Although Condélo is aware of the beliefs surrounding his albinism and their consequences, he is trapped in his marginality, hopelessly seeking refuge in dreams and solitude. Condélo expresses his simultaneous desire to belong and his acceptance of non-belonging:

---

28   Chevrier, *Le Lecteur d'Afriques*, 291.

> Si on était sûrs, Patience, qu'il y a un pays où pour vivre il faut laisser vivre, on serait partis tout de suite là-bas. C'est pour ça que je voulais m'instruire. Apprendre à connaître le monde entier, pour pouvoir choisir un coin où on ne verrait de sang versé. Mais personne n'a voulu m'aider'. (*Wirriyamu*, 120)

As *Wirriyamu* makes clear, individuals such as Condélo often feel alienated and powerless, perceiving their circumstances to be so unique that they cannot envisage a peer group with whom they can relate. The young Condélo is unhappy living in the village because he is bullied by the other children and, throughout his life, he experiences profound isolation and loneliness. Condélo is unable to cope with life within or outside of society, struggling constantly to come to terms with his exclusion. In contrast to the protagonists of the other novels, he fails to show any character development or any move towards addressing his situation in a positive way. This reflects the prevailing tone of the novel, which is generally one of despair and hopelessness, with only memories of a happier past.

Like Condélo, Sassine's Milo experiences bullying and isolation as a child. He recalls a specific incident to which he attaches great importance:

> Je ne suis devenu ce que je suis que par un matin. Les maîtres avaient organisé une sortie. A midi, nous devions nous baigner dans un petit lac naturel. [...] Quand je sortais de l'eau, mes habits avaient disparu et le groupe de filles arrivait. Je suis rentré à la maison, tout nu, tout grelottant, derrière ma classe, pendant que toute la ville me montrait du doigt. [...] Depuis ce jour, j'ai juré de ne plus pleurer. (*Mémoire*, 30)

The significance of these events is closely related to the symbolic nakedness of the albino body and the lack generally associated with it. The figurative lack of a skin leaves the young Milo vulnerable not only to the stares of other people, but also to their judgement. The removal of Milo's clothes functions as a reinforcement of his difference, exposing more of the albino body which marks him apart. However, unlike Condélo, in struggling to understand his marginality Milo comes to develop a strong sense of who he is, demonstrating that marginality can also be used constructively, to strategic advantage. As the following chapter will discuss in more detail, Milo's constant switching of identities and his manipulation of those around him reveals an assertion of individuality that permits him to maintain a sense of self. Although for others he is insignificant, 'un invisible, un rien' (*Mémoire*, 14), Milo's realisation of his position as outsider permits him to expose the workings of prejudice and judgement within society, and his constant critique of those around him underpins the narrative. Dynamic in his experience of 'in-betweenness', Milo is able to move easily and powerfully between different environments. In each, he acts in a way which enables him to gain the most from each situation. At the same time, his awareness of his alterity allows him to scrutinise his position and the reasons for it, and ultimately leads him to question the established social order.

It becomes evident that the encounter between dominant regulatory norms and the experience of those at the margins necessitates a continual process of negotiation. The relentless locating and re-locating of identity undertaken by the albino protagonists throughout the novels takes on significance in the light of Hall's discussion of identity. Hall suggests that there are two ways in which identity might be viewed. 'Identity as being' offers a sense of unity and commonality, in Hall's terms, 'defining cultural identity in terms of one, shared culture, a sort of collective "one true self", hiding inside the many other, more superficial or artificially imposed "selves".'[29] This position on identity initially appears attractive when considering albino identity, for it offers the potential for the person with albinism to be included on the basis of terms other than those of physical appearance. However, it also emerges as threatening for it homogenises, tending to hide not only those 'superficial and artificially imposed selves' of which Hall writes, but also those selves which are not considered 'acceptable' to society. This problematic is illustrated in both Sassine's *Wirriyamu* and Destremau's *Nègre blanc*. Sassine's Condélo is torn between a desire to share a sense of commonality with those around him and a simultaneous desire to be recognised for his difference. To the same end, Destremau's protagonist Samate does all he can to gain acceptance in the white community into which he is taken by Mafavuca, entailing as this does a process of cultural lactification:

---

29   Stuart Hall, 'Cultural Identity and Diaspora' in *Colonial Discourse & Postcolonial Theory: A Reader* ed. by Patrick Williams & Laura Chrisman (London: Harvester Wheatsheaf, 1993), 392–403 (393).

> Il sent qu'il vit une dichotomie insupportable, une double vie dont les éléments cohabitent mal en lui. L'existence dans ce cadre civilisé, ordonné, orienté vers un but, celui de préparer à y édifier sa place au soleil, c'est-à-dire s'y intégrer définitivement sans rémission selon une logique à laquelle il n'adhère pas, il la subit sans enthousiasme ni conviction. (*Nègre blanc*, 256)

However, this process only enforces the realisation of his difference. Samate later recalls that on the surface he may have appeared contented, but in truth he felt suffocated. Ultimately it is this sense of discomfort which persuades Samate to go in search of his own identity.

The second of Hall's suggestions, that identity be posited as a process of 'becoming', exposes the discontinuity in an individual's identity formation. Since an ever-changing identity that constantly re-positions itself is difficult to contain, the notion of 'identity as becoming' suggests a potentially powerful position from which to elude the need to categorise and homogenise.[30] On the level of individual identity, a parallel can be drawn with Destremau, Grainville and Sassine's portrayal of the marginalised albino as an individual involved in just such a process of improvisation. This act of becoming involves the complex negotiation of individuality and the definitions constructed or imposed by others, while at the same time operating as a challenge to dominant social and cultural norms. It is a process that confirms that the fragmented nature of albino subjectivity liberates it from restrictive binary definitions.

The centre/margin dichotomy that equated to a white/black binary was used during the colonial era to justify the colonisation of Africa. Ironically, the notion that the marginal should be included was used as the principal justification for the economic and political exploitation of colonialism, particularly under the French policies of the *mission civilisatrice*. This same notion has been used consistently by postcolonial critics to undermine the idea that a superior Western centre exists, deconstructing the claims of the colonisers to superiority. Although Destremau, Grainville and Sassine appear to subscribe to the notion of 'recentring the margins' in their reinscription of albinism in fiction, they continue to insist upon

---

30   Idem.

Inhabiting the Margins 139

the presence of boundaries that are not only intrinsic to the structure of the narrative, but also to the experiences of their protagonists. However one views the margin, whether as a firm divide or a space of agency, its presence cannot be denied. Yet, if the boundaries are to be re-drawn, the question arises as to how these will be defined and on what basis they will be constructed, for boundaries require categories of 'within' and 'without', the designation of those to be included and those to be excluded. Hence the question as to the extent to which we can escape categorisation, if at all, is raised again.

Said's approach to the analysis of boundaries is to accept their presence, but to dispute the importance we place upon them. He insists that, 'borders and barriers, which enclose us within the safety of familiar territory, can also become prisons, and are often defended beyond reason or necessity'.[31] Although Said focuses on the drawing of physical borders, his comments are equally applicable to more abstract imaginings of boundaries because, like physical borders, not only do constructed boundaries exclude certain individuals, but they also limit the experience of those whom they contain. The protagonists of *Nègre blanc*, *Le Tyran éternel* and *Wirriyamu* strive to escape the situations of alterity in which they find themselves and seek the attainment of a positive social status. However, these albino characters remain in the liminal or marginal sphere precisely because of the complexities that make impossible a reconciliation of the fragments of their identities. In these novels then, Destremau, Grainville and Sassine confirm Bhabha's notion of the margin as a place where identity can be performed and contested. Samate's progression from childhood to adulthood and consequent development of a sense of individual identity takes place on the margins of society, as does Milo's realisation of his exclusion that becomes a catalyst for his self affirmation. The margin is not simply represented in the novels as the negative border space to which all those who are deemed unacceptable to society are relegated, but instead it is posited as a space that permits the development and confirmation of albino identity.

31 Said, *Culture and Imperialism*, 252.

The following chapter explores the subversive potential of the figure of the albino in literature in terms of what Bhabha describes as 'a form of power exercised at the very limits of identity and authority'.[32] Just as the notion of the 'wild' confirms the need to secure the boundaries of civilisation, so the presence of the albino serves as a reminder of the precarious nature of the normative and all that is designated as acceptable. The following chapter will discuss the importance of power in the construction of identity through difference by exploring the various ways in which Destremau, Grainville and Sassine represent the associations between power, subordination and resistance. It will examine how, by constantly threatening to break down boundaries and binary oppositions from within, the albino body asserts a need to move beyond polarised positions on identity and dismantles constructions of the passive colonised body in favour of an unruly and resisting one.

32   Bhabha, *The Location of Culture*, 62.

CHAPTER 5

Power and Identity

The importance of power in the construction of identity through difference is central to the literary representation of albinism. Exploring that relationship further, this chapter examines the various ways in which Destremau, Grainville and Sassine represent the associations between violence and power, subordination and resistance. As previous chapters have demonstrated, the novels suggest that it is difficult to acknowledge the agency of the figure of the albino unless this is understood in terms of that individual's status as a victim. The paradox of marginalisation and empowerment discussed in the previous chapter locates the subversive potential of the albino in a form of power that is exercised at the very limits of identity. I pay particular attention to Sassine's novel *Mémoire d'une peau* in the first part of this chapter because of the complexity of the narrative, the remarkable negotiation of marginal identity undertaken by the protagonist Milo, and the different ways in which he attempts to assert power over others. Despite the often extreme nature of Milo's actions, I will suggest that the narrative of *Mémoire d'une peau* also delineates more covert and ambivalent forms of resistance to the dominant ideology that insistently positions the albino as a powerless other. In the second part of the chapter, the way in which the alterity of the albino and the subversive potential of this figure is portrayed in the four novels is explored in the context of a reclaiming and reinscribing of the albino body. I will argue that Destremau, Grainville and Sassine represent the figure of the albino in a way that highlights the need to move beyond polarised positions on identity towards a more flexible and inclusive position.

Violence and Power

Mémoire d'une peau, *Wirriyamu*, *Le Tyran éternel* and *Nègre blanc* are all imbued with a temporal awareness that firmly locates the personal experiences of the protagonists in a specific historical context, and the particular settings of the novels in colonial and postcolonial Africa signal a need to consider the power structures at work more closely. The narrative of Sassine's *Wirriyamu* unravels during the final years of colonial rule in Mozambique, where Portuguese colonisation lasted long after many European powers had granted independence to their colonies. The country only became independent on 25 June 1975 after the guerrilla force of the Liberation Front of Mozambique wrested control of the country from the Portuguese authorities. The violence of the last ten years of colonial rule in Mozambique is echoed in the narrative of *Wirriyamu*, which is set against the backdrop of the 1972 massacre of the villagers of Wirriyamu by the Portuguese. During the 'Wirriyamu Massacre', Portuguese soldiers were supposed to have killed over four hundred villagers in a village by that name. No village with that or any similar name in that area was ever proven to exist. Yet the stories of the Wirriyamu massacre and the search for the village of Wirriyamu made headlines all over the world for months.[1] In Sassine's novel, the threat posed by the Portuguese soldiers is expressed in their relentless march towards the village, an advance that has a sense of inevitability about it. This is compounded by the fragmentation of the book into small sections marking the progression of time over a period of three days. The population of Wirriyamu is depicted as trapped by the colonial situation, powerless as they are drawn inexorably towards the massacre. A constant threat of violence also manifests itself in the everyday acts of cruelty that are found throughout the narrative, carried out by the likes of the Portuguese Commander d'Arriaga who revels in his power over others. Beating the chief of the village in punishment for having allowed

---

[1] See 'The Persistant Empire', *Time Magazine*, Monday 23 December, 1973,<http://www.time.com/time/magazine/article/0,9171,910914-1,00.html> [Accessed 14 May 2010].

his villagers to run off, d'Arriaga takes apparent pleasure in the pain he inflicts on the man:

> Le commandant d'Arriaga leva la règle et frappa de toutes ses forces. D'un coup, elle éplucha les doigts de leur chair hachée. Il s'apprêtait encore à abaisser la règle lorsqu'un 'cipaye' vint en courant l'avertir que le téléphone sonnait. Il passa l'instrument de torture au secrétaire administratif. (103)

The matter-of-fact way in which the Commander deals with the punishment shows a complacency and lack of regard for his victims in his exercising of power over them. Said argues that colonialism manifested itself through the configurations of power that worked, and indeed still work, to control native lands and populations. He contends that ideas, culture and histories cannot be understood apart from configurations of power, and that the relationship between the Occident and the Orient is a relationship 'of power, of domination, of varying degrees of a complex hegemony'.[2] Sassine's *Wirriyamu* substantiates Said's argument, confirming that notions of white supremacy and racism constitute the power relationships and hierarchical structures that characterise the so-called 'civilising mission', and in doing so, draws out the inherent irony of the term. Commander d'Arriaga carries with him several pieces of paper on which are written what he terms the enlightened thoughts of Portugal's great men. The thoughts are certainly illuminating for the reader, but not in the way in which d'Arriaga takes them to be. Instead they reveal the thinking behind the Portuguese colonial mission. In an attempt to justify the violence he uses to control the colonised, d'Arriaga quotes Mousinko de Albuquerque: 'Lorsqu'une race forte conquiert un peuple inférieur, il est tout naturel qu'il y ait des abus' (148). D'Arriaga also cites Marcelo Caetano, a quotation which shows how the Portuguese viewed the colonised: 'L'indigène est un enfant, instinctivement méchant comme tous les enfants, mais comme eux, docile et sincère sur lequel le Blanc doit exercer une tutelle juste, humanitaire et civilisatrice' (149). Fanon refers to the commonplace colonial mythology of the infantile nature of the colonised in *Peau noire, masques blancs*, demonstrating that this infantilisation is a defensive reaction on the part of the coloniser,

---

2   Said, *Orientalism*, 5.

because the reality is that 'le nègre est un objet phobogène, anxiogène'.[3] Fanon uses several clinical cases to demonstrate that the colonised African generates great anxiety in the sub-consciousness of the coloniser.

Sassine's Condélo embodies the child-like immaturity assumed to be characteristic of the colonised in his naivety, his immature understanding of other people and childish relationship with his dog. However, Condélo is not the only victim in *Wirriyamu*. In his portrayal of the protagonist and other characters in the narrative as powerless in the face of the Portuguese onslaught, Sassine underscores the impact of events on the lives of the colonised. Old Ondo, warning Kabalango to leave the village, sums up the hopelessness of their situation and presages the violence that is to come:

> Etranger, vous avez déjà prouvé votre intelligence en rendant visite à Ondo. Alors, suivez ce conseil: continuez rapidement votre chemin car ce village est pourri jusqu'à ses arbres. Et lorsque vous entendrez derrière vous des cris de détresse et de mort, ne vous retournez pas. (77)

He correctly anticipates the violence which will ultimately destroy the village and the people of Wirriyamu in a brutal demonstration of colonial power.

By way of contrast to the colonial rule that shapes the world in which Sassine's *Wirriyamu* is set, dominance and control are embodied in the figure of the former dictator Houphouët-Boigny in Grainville's novel *Le Tyran éternel*. Having liberated Côte d'Ivoire from the colonising forces in 1960, the revolutionary Houphouët-Boigny ruled the country until his death in 1993. He was Africa's longest-serving head of state, having begun his political career as a left-wing nationalist under French colonial rule.[4] He maintained closer links with France than any other African leader and under his guidance Côte d'Ivoire became one of the most stable and prosperous states in Africa. However, it was only after thirty years of one-man, one-party rule, that he eventually conceded in 1990 to demands for free elections.[5]

---

3   Fanon, *Peau noire, masques blancs*, 96.
4   Pierre Nandjui, *Houphouët-Boigny: l'homme de la France en Afrique* (Paris: L'Harmattan, 1995), 56.
5   Marcel Amondji, *Félix Houphouët et la Côte d'Ivoire: L'envers d'une légende* (Paris: Karthala, 1985), 12–13.

Narrated by the deceased Houphouët-Boigny, Grainville's novel is an ironic portrayal of a leader obsessed with power and grandeur, whom Grainville describes as typical of the postcolonial dictators who stepped into the power vacuum left by the colonisers. Achille Mbembe comments: 'A l'ombre de la postcolonie ont grandi des monstres.'[6] Perpetuating the oppression suffered under colonialism, dictators grew out of the challenge faced by African countries attempting to establish nationhood in the wake of colonial rule. In *Le Tyran éternel*, the dictator-like character of Houphouët-Boigny imagines himself to be a God, governing Yamoussoukro from above: 'Je suis le Sage de Yamoussoukro. Mais aussi le Sang. Ainsi j'ai tenu jusqu'au bout... à bout portant. Personne n'a réussi à me renverser' (12). The reference to the blood of Yamoussoukro recalls the repeated use of body imagery throughout *Le Tyran éternel*. The image of Houphouët-Boigny's blood coursing through the veins of the city is an interesting one, because it expresses the close personal involvement of the dictator in its development – and that of Côte d'Ivoire – and at the same time reveals any threat to the city to be a personal threat to him. The particular nature of his interest in the city, and consequently its security, is articulated in his despotism, which prescribes the way in which the city of Yamoussoukro and its inhabitants function. Such is his control that the supremacy of Houphouët-Boigny remains unquestioned until his son returns to challenge him.

Destremau's *Nègre blanc* is also set against a background of tyranny – the historical backdrop to the novel is that of the 1962 Civil War in Mozambique – although in this novel we witness a shift in power taking place on a personal scale rather than a national one. Samate's childhood is barely touched by the war unfolding beyond the bounds of the forest where he spends his formative years. Only Mafavuca is aware of the ongoing war and he is far from concerned as he observes the planes flying overhead. There is a sense that the forest provides the family with security, distancing them from the events of the war. Even as an ex-soldier who knows the danger of war, Mafavuca can watch events unfolding with a sense of detachment.

---

6 Achille Mbembe, 'Désordres, résistances et productivité' in *Politique Africaine*, 39 (1991), 7–24 (7).

In the same disengaged way, violence forms the backdrop to the life of the protagonist of Sassine's *Mémoire d'une peau*. Although there is no specific mention of where the action of the novel takes place, allusions in the narrative to the ongoing *coup d'état*, arbitrary mass arrests and corruption, and bureaucrats and politicians who are defined by their inertia, suggest that it is Guinea.[7] On 2 October 1958, Guinea proclaimed itself a sovereign and independent republic, with Sékou Touré as President. Touré's early presidency was markedly leftist as he attempted to forge a socialist revolution through the early years of independence. However, as his policies failed, Touré adopted an increasingly centralised rule and Guinea became a one-party dictatorship, with a closed economy and little tolerance for human rights or the freedom of expression. Political opposition was ruthlessly suppressed and, although originally acknowledged for his cross-ethnic nationalism, over time Touré came to draw solely on his own Malinké ethnic group to fill positions of power. The regime alleged plots and conspiracies against Touré, torturing and executing opponents, and imprisoning thousands more in Soviet-style prison gulags. Meanwhile, more than a million Guineans were driven into exile. Touré's paranoia irreparably damaged relations both with neighbouring African states and foreign nations, increasing Guinea's isolation and devastating its economy. Touré and the PDG remained in power until his death on 3 April 1984. While some remember the president as a great pan-Africanist who attempted to unite Africa and Africans worldwide, it is difficult to ignore the realities of Camp Boiro and the economic, social and cultural legacies of his regime. Sassine recalls: 'Touré always lived in ideological confusion; for this, we in Guinea loved him or hated him. He had his partisans and opponents. Most of the partisans were following him out of fear'.[8]

As in Destremau's novel, references to the violence taking place are rarely elaborated upon, but are woven into the narrative in such a way

---

7   Mahmoud Bah, *Construire la Guinée: Après Sékou Touré* (Paris: L'Harmattan, 1990), 5–31.
8   Manthia Diawara, *In Search of Africa* (Cambridge, MA: Harvard University Press, 1998) 48.

that they are barely noticeable, built into the fabric of the world in which the characters live. The violent events of the *coup d'état* have become part of Milo's everyday life. Although not causally related to the hostility of the *coup d'état*, violence also operates on another level in *Mémoire d'une peau*. Milo's own violent behaviour takes many forms and is most notably translated into his acts of killing. Through the course of the narrative Milo discloses that he has killed six people, but suggests that there have been others, admitting, 'J'ai plusieurs fois tué' (*Mémoire*, 44). The violence of his acts is excessive, but the reasoning behind them brings the reader to understand that these are not solely acts of arbitrary killing, but of revenge, as they are all directly or indirectly related to his albinism. Milo remembers how the Headteacher mercilessly teased him at school and made him an object of ridicule. In revenge for this and his intrusion into Milo's family life by sleeping with his mother, Milo kills the Headteacher's daughter:

> Deux ans après sa mort, le directeur de l'école était dans ton lit. Je me suis bouché les oreilles. Le lendemain j'étais chez lui. Il faisait noir, j'avais poussé le portail. Il était au ciné avec sa femme. J'ai vu leur fillette. Dans les cinq ans. J'ai pris un gros caillou... (*Mémoire*, 32)

Milo's loathing of his mother's lovers, whom he perceives to be a threat to his family, is summed up in one sentence: 'Maman, je voulais te garder pour moi seul et pour papa' (35). Milo's accounts of his acts are brief, which is significant, for it becomes clear that it is not the act of killing that is important to Milo, but the reason for killing, which he elaborates at great length throughout the novel. His violence fulfils his desire for revenge against those who teased him as a child, the teachers who bullied him, and people like the Andréa family who offer him little respect.

The violence of Milo's acts operates as a reassertion of power against those who have attempted to disempower him. However, it becomes clear that Milo's violence results only in the seemingly unnecessary death of his victims and meets with the passivity of people such as his mother, in the face of which his violence has little meaning. Looking through her photograph album, Milo's mother comments, 'mon album de photos est un cimetière' (34). However, she does not apportion blame, but instead gives a passive response in her reluctant acceptance or denial of Milo's violent acts, telling him only that she fears for him. As a child, Milo recalls having broken the wings of birds his father brought home for him, and remembers having caused other animals suffering: 'Je faisais souffrir de petites bêtes innocentes. Je voulais un reproche, un blâme, un châtiment. Je cherchais la différence entre le bien et le mal' (64). Just as he was not taught the difference between right and wrong as a child, the line between the two seems to remain blurred for the adult Milo too. There is no indication in the narrative that Milo has been punished for his acts of killing, nor any suggestion that people other than his mother and father are aware that Milo has committed these crimes. Milo's violence does not result in any more than an immediate sense of power over his victims, who for so long exercised their authority over him. However, his murderous acts provide him with personal satisfaction, for they are both a means of appeasing the little voice in his head and allow him to take personal vengeance for what he perceives to be the wrong-doings of his victims.

Thus, power and violence, in their different forms, are found on both personal and national levels in *Mémoire d'une peau*, and although they are not always directly linked in the novel, it is possible to draw parallels between them. The association between power and violence is more overt in *Mémoire d'une peau* than in the other three narratives, perhaps because in Sassine's novel there is a constantly shifting balance of power. Milo refers to shifts in power on a national level, referring to 'l'ancien régime' and 'les périodes d'arrestations massives' (134). So, the dictatorial power exercised by the leaders of the country is met with violence from those carrying out the *coup d'état* which forms the backdrop to the action of the novel. Yet, it also becomes apparent that there is a constant shifting of power on a personal level as Milo manipulates people and situations to his advantage, and demonstrates that it is still possible to exercise power from the margins, albeit an often-fleeting sense of authority over another.

Networks of Resistance

Whereas Milo fails to achieve power over others through violence, he successfully uses other means of recuperating power, which most often manifest themselves in various forms of resistance. Resistance is generally understood to stand in opposition to power and this is usually a power held by an elite that use oppressive means by which to secure authority. However, modes of resistance are not always clearly delineated in Sassine's novel, perhaps because like power, resistance is not static but exists in many forms. It is important to draw out this complexity, in the light of the network of interwoven threads of power and resistance in *Mémoire d'une peau*.

In their study of power and resistance, in which they explore themes of identity, embodiment and colonialism, Sharp et al. critique orthodox accounts of power, domination and resistance. They suggest that a Foucauldian perspective on the many social, political and cultural relations of power between individuals and groups might be a more productive way of addressing this relationship.[9] Foucault's formulation of power acknowledges that neither dominating power nor resisting power is total, but instead that they are fragmentary and inconsistent, and neither can exist without the other. As Sharp et al. observe, 'No moment of domination can be completely free of relations of resistance and likewise no moment of resistance, in whatever form, is entirely segregated from relations of dominance.'[10]

Resistance operates overtly in *Mémoire d'une peau* as Milo openly criticises different aspects of the society in which he lives and works. He describes the tentacular bureaucracy of his workplace:

---

9   Joanne P. Sharp et al., 'Entanglements of Power: Geographies of Domination/Resistance' in Joanne P. Sharp, Paul Routledge, Chris Philo and Ronan Paddison (eds), *Entanglements of Power: Geographies of Domination/Resistance* (London: Routledge, 2000), 1–43.
10 Ibid., 20.

> La pieuvre était déjà bien en place avec ses bras de la bureaucratie métastasante du socialisme de l'ancien régime, sa grosse tête globuleuse et immobile de l'inertie tropicale, les ventouses de ses secrétaires ondulantes. (20–1)

The metaphor of the octopus here expresses the all-consuming power of the ancien régime's legacy of bureaucracy and Milo's sense of frustration at the inertia of the people he works with. Milo's use of the adjective 'métastasante' suggests the cancerous nature of such bureaucracy. He condemns his male peers, whom he finds 'trop petits ou trop gros dans leur corps, leurs gestes et surtout leurs opinions' (15), and criticises women about whom he remarks, 'les femmes se classaient en deux catégories: les bonnes et les belles. Les unes perdent vite leur vertu et les autres leur parfum' (19). Milo's condemnation of the society in which he lives is enduring, aimed not at any one establishment or individual, but instead fragmented as he targets issues that have an immediate and usually adverse effect on his own life. At work he is frustrated by the inanity of his job – he has come under physical and psychological attack on many occasions by his male peers – and as we shall discuss later in this chapter, he is aware that his weakness for women leaves him particularly vulnerable.

On a more subtle level, resistance manifests itself in behaviour that undermines the structures and strategies of domination in Milo's world. These subtle forms of resistance can be seen most clearly in the form of humour, an insistent critique of society and a play on the multiplicity of meaning. This humorous critique is a form of symbolic resistance consistent with what Scott terms the 'weapons of the weak', which he describes as 'tools of indirect opposition to the dominator'.[11] Scott illustrates his argument with reference to the master/slave dialectic proposed by Hegel. For Hegel, the master is a consciousness that can only define itself in relation to the slave's consciousness:

---

11 James C. Scott, *Weapons of the Weak: Everyday Forms of Peasant Resistance* (New Haven: Yale University Press, 1985), 29.

Power and Identity

> The consciousness for-the-Master is not an independent but a dependent, consciousness. Thus he is not certain of existence-for-self as the truth; rather, his truth is the inessential consciousness and the inessential action of the latter [the slave].[12]

Among the many implications of the master-slave dialectic is the idea of reciprocity or mutual dependence between master and slave, rather than a blanket opposition of dominance to subordination. The slave ironically shares in the master's power because the master defines himself only in opposition to the slave, that is, the master needs the slave in order to legitimate his comparative privilege.

Fanon takes issue with the problems Hegel's master-slave dialectic encounters in its translation into a post-colonial context. The Hegelian dialectic suggests a relationship between the concrete and the abstract, subject and object, master and slave. However, Fanon criticises Hegel's master-slave dialectic because he considers it to be an unequal power relationship. In *Peau noire, masques blancs*, Fanon revises the dialectic to suggest that it underestimates the white master's dominance over black slaves in Africa and Europe:

> Nous espérons avoir montré que le maître ici diffère essentiellement de celui décrit par Hegel. Chez Hegel il y a réciprocité, ici le maître se moque de la conscience de l'esclave. Il ne réclame pas la reconnaissance de ce dernier, mais son travail.[13]

Scott too indicates that the slave is not in a position, within the unequal power dynamics of the relationship between the master and the slave, to refuse to work or to directly criticise his or her owner without the risk of serious consequences. Thus, Scott suggests, the forms of resistance used must be more subtle, an undercurrent of ideological resistance beneath a surface of compliance.[14]

12 Georg Wilhelm Friedrich Hegel, *Phenomenology of Spirit*, translated by A.V. Miller (Oxford: Oxford University Press, 1981), 61. Discussed in Robert C. Solomon, *In the Spirit of Hegel: a Study of G.W.F. Hegel's Phenomenology of Spirit* (New York: Oxford University Press, 1983), 318–40.
13 Fanon, *Peau noire, masques blancs*, 179.
14 Scott, *Weapons of the* Weak, 31–3.

The subtle forms of resistance at work in *Mémoire d'une peau* are directed at the practices by which Milo is marginalised, serving to critique the structures which elevate others to positions of superiority. Sassine's novel offers a biting analysis of the world from the margins by using humour as an oblique critique of those individuals and groups whom he perceives to hold power over him, and a condemnation of all that they deem acceptable. Just as discussion of the stereotype earlier in *Enduring Negativity* noted that its power is dependent on its audience, it becomes evident that humour too depends upon a number of variables including its contextual circumstance. The same joke, caricature or image can be employed as a comedy-creating exercise, used ironically as a sign of shared recognition or friendship, or used with hostile intent, depending upon who it is shared with and at whom it is directed.

Milo addresses his humour to the readers, confiding in them throughout the novel. Sassine's novels were published in both France and Africa and he directs his fictional work at a mixed audience, addressing his readership by referring to specific events, places and cultural markers. Milo mentions Jacques Chirac, as well as the Mauritanian cinematographer Med Hondo whose documentaries were highly critical of imperialist attitudes, and refers to 'le Bembeya Jazz' (*Mémoire*, 75), a Guinean band known for its Afro-pop which was particularly successful in the early days of Guinean independence. As Milo confides in the reader, he assumes that the readership will concur with him, agreeing with his views which expose the assumptions and failings of the society in which he lives. In reality the mixed readership will mean that there is no certainty that this will be the case, but Sassine's narrative technique is successful in drawing the reader into an intimate and even collaboratory relationship with his protagonist Milo.

Milo's acerbic, yet perceptive remarks echo the tone of the narrative as a whole. He describes dinner with the Andréa couple:

> Hier, nous étions chez les Andréa, un couple de sexagénaires malheureux pour n'avoir jamais connu la pauvreté [...] Je ne les aimais pas du tout. Les Andréa me le rendaient bien, en se servant de mon épouse qu'ils avaient 'adoptée' et qu'ils appelaient Mimi. [...] Et puis cet inévitable jeu de ping-pong hebdomadaire dans lequel je tenais le rôle de balle. (10–11)

Milo sums up his position in just one sentence, using the imagery of the ping pong ball to convey his frustration. He is forced to continually defend himself from his wife on one side and the Andréas on the other, a situation which Milo finds tedious and only endures so that he might have his Mondays to himself. At the same meal, Milo's description of the soup is another example of his sardonic criticism:

> Avec de la viande musclée d'une vache ayant traversé deux océans à la nage, ou avec un poisson des eaux pour apprendre à marcher? Avec trop de piment ou trop d'oignons? Cela dépendait des dimanches. [...] Ce n'était ni la vache aquatique, ni le poisson-piéton. Peut-être un poulet s'il n'y avait les trois cuisses qui flottaient. (12)

The idea of a three-legged chicken, a walking fish or a swimming cow is ridiculous. However, given the preceding conversation at the dinner table, it becomes evident that Milo's reflection on the soup is a contemplation of the fascination with which he is met because of his failure to 'fit' into any designated category. Milo's sarcastic humour is a tool with which he attempts to reclaim power by highlighting and criticising the very practices by which he is marginalised as a person with albinism. Unsurprisingly, the narrative implies that those in privileged positions who are the butt of Milo's sarcasm do not find it amusing. His humour is met with silence or, in the case of the meal with the Andréa couple, the conversation changes direction. Elsewhere in the narrative the sarcastic remarks are addressed to the reader and consequently the reaction of those to whom they are directed is unseen.

Susanne Reichl and Mark Stein's study of humour in postcolonial fiction supports the argument that Milo's wit is a means of promoting agency.[15] Drawing on Freud's understanding of the joke as a socially acceptable form of attack and Boskin's argument that humour's particularity lies in its 'elastic polarity', Reichl and Stein suggest that laughter is a device that is 'self-consciously employed and strategically positioned in postcolonial textual constructions, or an effect elicited by these'.[16] Their analysis draws particularly on Joseph Boskin's suggestion that:

---

15 Susanne Reichl and Mark Stein (eds), *Cheeky Fictions: Laughter and the Postcolonial* (Amsterdam: Rodopi, 2005), 1–27.
16 Ibid., 10.

> [Humour] can operate for and against, deny or affirm, oppress or liberate. On the one hand, it reinforces pejorative images; on the other, it facilitates the inversion of such stereotypes. Just as it has been utilized as a weapon of insult and persecution, so, too, has humor been implemented as a device of subversion and protest.[17]

Thus Reichl and Stein suggest that humour is a means of recuperating power. Indeed, although superficially amusing, Milo's observations function as a broader critique of the society in which he lives. Douglas describes the subversive potential of humour as 'A victorious tilting of uncontrol against control [...] an image of the levelling of hierarchy, the triumph of intimacy over formality, or unofficial values over official ones.'[18] This definition serves equally to describe Sassine's *Mémoire d'une peau*, such is the tone of the novel. Milo openly criticises those who hold positions of respect in the community, from the mayor 'un gros con qui aimait déjà imiter la voix des autres avant d'être élu' (42), to the rich white tourists, 'leurs femmes grimées en mannequins boudinés, leur peau qui leur faisait mal parce qu'elles ne grillaient pas assez vite au soleil de leur Afrique' (74). This last rather pointed comment brings to mind the vulnerability of Milo's albino skin to damage from the sun.

Milo refuses to accept hypocrisy or the wearing of masks, preferring to associate with individuals who do not put up a façade. His friend capitaine Kali is just one example:

> Du balcon me parvenait une musique antillaise et j'apercevais la longue silhouette du capitaine Kali. Il dansait tout seul. Il n'avait jamais d'état d'âme. Je l'aimais bien. [...] Celui-là n'était pas un compliqué. Une femme à qui il offrait tout et qu'il battait à mort une fois par mois. (66)

Milo's criticism is never directed at people such as capitaine Kali, but instead at those who pretend to be what they are not. Speaking of his encounter with a prostitute for example, he comments: 'Je n'ai jamais aimé les baiseuses

---

17   Joseph Boskin, *Rebellious Laughter: People's Humor in American Culture* (Syracuse, NY: Syracuse University Press, 1997) 38 cited in Reichl and Stein, 11.
18   Mary Douglas, *Implicit Meanings: Essays in Anthropology* (London: Routledge, 1975), 98.

Power and Identity

professionnelles, celles qui s'allument dès que vous glissez une pièce dans leur fente' (48). This statement is typical of Milo's contemptuous humour as he offers his scornful, but piercing analysis of the people around him and their motives.

Not only does Milo's remark expose the purely economic motives of the prostitute, but it also reveals his general attitude towards women, which is openly negative and always disrespectful. His means of escape from the reality of living with albinism manifests itself in his womanising; an objectification of women that recurs throughout the narrative in many forms. Expressing the lack of meaning in his encounters with women and exposing his misanthropic tendencies, Milo remarks:'Je fais la chasse aux femmes comme d'autres sont chasseurs de lapins ou d'éléphants, de diplômes ou de rêves' (*Mémoire*, 15). He describes his womanising as a quest, boasting about his numerous lovers:

> J'ai commencé par les prénoms du calendrier. Je me disais que parmi tous ces saints noms, quelqu'une pourrait m'aider à comprendre... [...] J'ai épuisé la liste des saintes. De A à Z. Plusieurs fois. (135)

The lack of meaning in Milo's relationships is reflected in his promise to his wife that he will be faithful, which he finds he is unable to keep. It becomes apparent then that humour functions to subvert in *Mémoire d'une peau*, as Milo reveals and challenges the attitudes of those who believe themselves to be superior to him. The validity of their mind-set is challenged and the reader is led to question the ways in which Milo is marginalised as an individual who does not fit the mould, and the motives behind this.

Milo's humour is often self-deprecatory, a self-reflexive humour that is made explicit by the very nature of the first person narrative. He describes how his appointment to the position of assistant to the press attaché encouraged him to better himself so he aspired to shouting, giving orders and organising those around him. However, the reality of his working life is rather different. It is dull and empty. Milo's remark 'J'étais payé pour faire le tailleur de papier' (21) demonstrates a propensity in the novel to say a great deal in very few words. Despite the grand office he occupies and the apparent status confirmed by his three secretaries, Milo's job is the epitome of mundanity. It becomes a metaphor for the hollowness that exists beneath the fragile façade of principles and values of the hierarchical society in which he lives, the very values that ensure Milo's constant marginalisation as a person with albinism where outward appearances are all-important. Realising the pointless nature of his job and the absence of any pleasure in his family life, and in the light of the lack of certainty that follows his mother's revelation that he was adopted, Milo comments, 'Donc, je n'avais rien. Rien du tout. J'aurais pu descendre du ciel ou sortir de la terre comme ça, comme une plante, une simple trace de la vie, un spermatozoïde qui se promène...' (40). In this way, Milo focuses his commentary upon himself, analysing his situation in a humorous, but critical way.

This re-focusing is particularly interesting in the light of Nancy Walker's analysis of humour, which suggests that laughing at one's own situation and shortcomings is a way of diminishing their importance and overcoming them. Walker indicates that it is also a way of cleansing them of the pejorative connotations imposed by the dominant culture and that by this means that they can be turned into strengths.[19] Milo's self-deprecatory humour complicates the power dynamic in *Mémoire d'une peau* because as the joker he appears to surrender control by emphasising his own inadequacies and therefore implicitly acknowledging the superiority of others over him. However, in light of Walker's analysis of self-reflexive humour as a tool of resistance, it becomes evident that the surrender of power in *Mémoire d'une peau* is an illusion. In his commentary, Milo is able to preserve a sense of self that is independent from his construction as other by the very people whose way of life and mindset he critiques, and in his use of irony and satire he exposes the attitudes that function to marginalise people with albinism.

Milo's self-contemplative narration also reveals him to be an individual who constantly questions his situation, as he attempts to view himself as others see him and asserts his desire to succeed. Reflecting on his childhood, for example, Milo describes how he felt the need for acceptance: 'Je ne

---

19 Nancy Walker, *A Very Serious Thing: Women's Humor and American Culture* (Minneapolis: University of Minnesota Press, 1988), xxiii.

retrouvais un peu de fraternité qu'en courant derrière le ballon dans lequel je tapais comme un fou. On prit pour un don ce qui n'était qu'agressivité défoulée et volonté de me faire accepter' (25). However, Milo's desire to be included was continually thwarted by the bullying of his peers and the jokes they played on him, which served only to mark him further apart. Ngũgĩ wa Thiong'o suggests that an articulation of resistance requires an examination of how we participate in our own oppression.[20] The process of 'decolonising the mind', to use Ngũgĩ's terminology, is founded upon the capacity to think oneself out of the position of 'Other'.[21] He proposes that intellectual awareness, critical self-reflection, and self-analysis hold the potential for transforming the life of the oppressed. Benita Parry concurs, suggesting that those individuals who are othered, excluded, or discriminated against have to realise their own solutions.[22] Indeed, the adult Milo is dynamic in resisting categorisation by others, instead actively defining and redefining his own identity: 'Je m'appelle Milo Kan. Je le répète trois fois comme une prière, avant de me lever tout doucement' (7). The development of Milo from a vulnerable child into an assertive adult results from his constant reflection on his own position and the society in which he lives, and the realisation that only by asserting his individuality can he overcome the threat of definition from without. As an adult, although Milo is actually relatively integrated, his own actions serve to ensure his marginality. He no longer simply desires inclusion, but instead claims a space outside the society which excludes him, a space from which he asserts his agency. As a consequence, he does not think himself out of the position of other, as Ngũgĩ suggests, but instead he actively constructs his otherness.

In *Peau noire, masques blancs* Fanon declares that the colonised are not victims, but rather that they are responsible for themselves as individuals within the structures in which they live: 'La densité de l'Histoire

20 Ngũgĩ wa Thiong'o, *Decolonizing the Mind: The Politics of Language in African Literature* (London: James Curry, 1986), 1–16.
21 Ibid., 15.
22 Benita Parry, 'Resistance Theory/Theorising Resistance or Two Cheers for Nativism' in *Colonial Discourse/Postcolonial Theory* ed. by F. Barker, P. Hulme, & M. Inversen (Manchester: Manchester University, 1994), 172–96 (196).

ne détermine aucun de mes actes. Je suis mon propre fondement.'²³ Fanon suggests that the colonised are made to feel silenced, and must therefore begin questioning and become critically engaged in contending dominant discourse. The first person narrative of *Mémoire d'une peau* shows Milo to be constantly questioning his own acts and critiquing those of others. His self-questioning stance functions as a means of reclaiming a sense of self as he asserts a self-defined identity over that imposed from without. His lack of regard for other people and a complete lack of any sense of collective responsibility further reinforce this, for his relationships with those around him, if they can be called 'relationships', serve only to isolate him further as an individual.

The positive consequences of Samate's self-examination in Destremau's *Nègre blanc* also support Fanon's assertion that the colonised must question their situation. Samate considers his circumstances critically, comparing his personal experience with that of the slaves in Harriet Beecher-Stowe's 1852 abolitionist novel *Uncle Tom's Cabin*: 'Comme eux, il est un transplant vivant loin de sa maison, de sa terre mythique à force d'avoir été désirée et sublimée, vivant une vie qu'il n'a pas choisie' (259). *Uncle Tom's Cabin* treats slavery as a central theme and the novel dramatises the harsh reality of slavery, although it has since been criticised for its condescending racial descriptions and stereotypes, and the passive way in which characters such as Uncle Tom accept their fate.²⁴ Unlike Uncle Tom and his fellow slaves, Samate constantly examines the situation in which he finds himself, eventually choosing to take his future into his own hands:

> Je ne suis pas un garçon comme les autres, tu le sais, et je ne peux espérer une vie conforme à celle des autres. [...] Mafavuca, je veux devenir chanteur. Je sens que c'est seulement dans la musique que je ferai quelque chose. (286)

---

23   Fanon, *Peau noire, masques blancs*, 187.
24   Richard Yarborough, 'Strategies of Black Characterization in Uncle Tom's Cabin and the Early Afro-American Novel' in Eric J. Sundquist (ed.), *New Essays on Uncle Tom's Cabin* (Cambridge: Cambridge University Press, 1993), 45–85.

Power and Identity

Realising that he will never find belonging in his adoptive father's world, Samate draws on his experiences and the relationships he has formed during his lifetime as a child living in his native village, in the marginal space of the forest and later in his adoptive father's town, to create a world of his own in which he can be accepted for who he is:

> Samate dirige son groupe de chanteurs constitué principalement par ses condisciples, qu'ils soient blancs ou noirs. Il commence ses tournées dans le sud du continent puis en Afrique de l'Ouest. Avant de partir pour l'Europe il publie un premier album composé de deux disques, baptisés bien sûr 'Mafavuca'. (286)

While Destremau's *Nègre blanc* depicts Samate coming to a realisation of his situation, as reflected in the linear structure of the novel, Sassine's *Mémoire d'une peau* is more complex. As I have already signalled, the narrative of *Mémoire d'une peau* unfolds on three levels: the novel *Mémoire d'une peau* with Milo as the protagonist, the romantic novel Milo attempts to write, and the letters exchanged between Milo and his lovers Rama and Christian, which reflect retrospectively on the events we have witnessed as readers. Because of these multiple layers of narration, it is possible to trace different perspectives on the same events in the novel such as Milo's first encounter with Rama:

> Abou la fit asseoir à notre table [...]. C'est ainsi que je fis votre connaissance, Rama. (*Mémoire*, 50)

> Elle venait vers notre table. Je m'étais déjà désintéressé d'elle. Sa démarche nerveuse, ton regard oblique. (157)

The complexity of the narrative is further reinforced by the recurrent conflict between past, present and future as Sassine's manipulation of time and use of flashback reveals the immense and continuing impact of Milo's childhood on his adult life. Sassine uses this technique of palimpsestic overlap throughout *Mémoire d'une peau*, a convolution of the narrative that not only complicates the reading of the novel, but is also associated with another tendency in the narrative, that is the layering of meanings discussed in Chapter 2 of *Enduring Negativity*.

This layering can be seen in the direct contradictions that reveal a manipulation by Milo of the meanings attributed to his albino body. *Mémoire d'une peau* is full of instances which demonstrate a manipulation of meaning, but the significance of these only becomes evident as they are considered in relation to discourse. Milo tells us: 'J'avais une sale gueule et je maudis une fois de plus l'accident qui m'avait défiguré en albinos' (70). However, as we have seen, he takes advantage of his albinism to play on the sensibilities of a group of foreign women: 'Je leur apprenais à s'émouvoir sur ma condition' (74). The passage exposes the way in which Milo manipulates those around him, convincing the women that he is a rare specimen, in need of protection. However, the play on their emotions is only further evidence of the platitudes that permit such beliefs to exist in the first place.

Milo often uses the stigma of his albinism to highlight his difference and to manipulate people to his advantage. Individuals with albinism have long taken advantage of their marked difference from those around them. Yellowman, a Jamaican reggae star of the 1980s, and Salif Keita, a singer and song-writer from Mali who appears as a character in Grainville's *Le Tyran éternel*, are just two individuals who have taken advantage of their distinctive appearance to facilitate their success in the music industry. As Bhabha argues:

> The question of identification is never the affirmation of a pre-given identity, never a self-fulfilled prophecy – it is always the production of an 'image' of identity and the transformation of the subject in assuming that image… identity is never an *a priori*, nor a finished product; it is only ever the problematic process of access to an 'image' of totality.[25]

Milo's experience of constructing identity is neither as positive nor as straightforward as Salif Keita's. However, the fact that he enacts change is important because in doing so, he demonstrates that he is not willing to be the passive recipient of an identity imposed from without, but instead, that he is actively engaged in the construction of his own unique identity.

---

25   Homi Bhabha, 'The Managed Identity – Foreword: Remembering Fanon' in Frantz Fanon, *Black Skin, White Masks* (London: Pluto Press, 1986), xvi–xvii.

Power and Identity

A similar claiming of identity is represented in Grainville's *Le Tyran éternel*. Until his meeting with Salif Keita, Alpha expresses his albinism in the same terms as those by which he is defined by others, but in the company of the other people with albinism, his skin serves as an outward sign of his shared experience with Salif. The same sense of understanding is shared between Milo and Sadou in Sassine's *Mémoire d'une peau*. Milo tells the deaf-mute Sadou of his love for Rama and Christian:

> – Mon frère, je suis amoureux. Tu t'en fiches, tu n'entends pas. Comment te faire comprendre que je viens de connaître l'amour, le vrai... Il s'était concentré sur le mouvement de mes lèvres.
> – Je cherche à oublier une femme et un homme...
> Il hochait la tête. Il comprenait. Avec lui je savais que ce n'était ni la langue, ni les bruits qui rapprochaient les hommes, mais la sympathie, mais la commune expérience, mais surtout la douleur, la passion. (154)

Although Sadou and Milo recognise the impossibility of their unique situations, their sense of shared understanding means that where once they were excluded, now others are excluded from their dialogue. So it becomes apparent that the manipulation of meaning found in the novels, and particularly in *Mémoire d'une peau*, has a situational logic to it. Milo manipulates the way in which he speaks and presents himself differently depending on whom he is speaking to. This is also the case in Grainville's *Le Tyran éternel* when Alpha meets Salif Keita. Theirs is a mode of resistance which operates on a micrological level and serves to undermine dominant ideologies. It is a means of resisting the values and ideas which ensure that prevailing social relations are perceived by most members of society to be natural, or are not seen at all.

The layering of different sets of values and ideas in the narratives is related to the climate of duplicity found in Sassine's novel in particular. In *Mémoire d'une peau*, the society in which Milo lives is characterised by deception and double-values. Milo's description of Hadja illustrates this most clearly. He describes her as 'La trentaine, jolie et intouchable officiellement' (43). However, Milo describes how he watched his father and Hadja one night and realised that her public face was very different from her private one:

> J'observais la tyrannie, la dissimulation, la discrète existence parallèle d'une femme qui ne sortait que voilée et dont il était interdit de serrer la main. [...] Je regardais en me disant que dans quelques heures elle serait la Hadja, la Grande, la Vertueuse et j'ai commencé à m'étonner que les hommes et les femmes se cachent pour s'aimer simplement. (44)

The contrast between public and private, official and unofficial is exposed in Hadja's wearing of the veil. The *hijab* worn by Hadja has been considered alternately as a symbol of oppression or a sign of piety, modesty and purity. For the Muslim woman, wearing the hijab fulfils the requirement of Islam for modesty in both men and women and the hope is that both will then be evaluated for intelligence and skills instead of looks and sexuality. A woman who covers herself is said to be concealing her sexuality, but at the same time expressing her femininity. By day Sassine's Hadja, whose name confirms that she has made a pilgrimage to Mecca, plays the role of the devoutly religious woman who conforms by covering her head. However, beneath the veil is the woman that Milo knows intimately, a woman who longs for sexual fulfilment and needs love. The passage demonstrates the disparity between expectation and actuality, at the same time revealing the possibility of manipulating the boundary between the two. Hadja uses her veil in much the same way that Milo uses his albinism; as a means of manipulating the way in which others perceive her and exaggerating the characteristics by which she can gain the most advantage at any one time.

Milo's relationship with Rama exposes and challenges perceptions of what is permissible. Looking at the woman he is holding in his arms, Milo reflects on their relationship:

> Je la regardai, sa belle peau cuivrée sur ma peau de nègre blanc de vitiligo, de lumière répugnante et j'avais envie de pleurer de bonheur, moi l'albinos, sans enfance, sans père ni mère, états civils truqués, ayant grandi parmi des funambules 'nuiteux' et repoussants. [...] Mais j'étais en train de baiser avec l'une des plus belles étrangères de la ville... (111)

When Rama first appears in the novel, walking into the bar in which Milo and his friends are drinking, she is described as a glamorous foreign woman who is holidaying in the area with her husband. All the men in the bar admire her, but none dare approach her. Despite the appearance of his albino body, the associations of his albinism and his dubious social status, of all the men in the bar Milo is the one who succeeds in seducing Rama. Perhaps because Rama too is an outsider, Milo finds he can relate to her. He does not worry that Rama is married to Christian. In fact, this makes the situation more appealing to Milo and he will eventually consider himself friends, and have sexual relationships with, both husband and wife.

Destremau's *Nègre blanc* also portrays a protagonist who is empowered by doing the unexpected. Samate's eventual success as a singer, which ultimately confirms his integration, is unforeseen. There is no mention of his ability to sing throughout the narrative of *Nègre blanc*, yet it is Samate's talent that ultimately enables him to celebrate his albino identity rather than restraining or altering it so that he might be included within more acceptable groups in society. In the same way, Alpha's succession to the rule of Yamoussoukro at the culmination of *Le Tyran éternel* represents a reversal of power as the once marginalised Alpha – who was not only socially, but physically excluded – is re-incorporated into society in a new role. We learn from his mother that:

> Houphouët n'aurait jamais voulu que l'enfant survécût [...]. Rien ne devait diminuer ses chances aux élections et sa capacité de garder le pouvoir. Il n'aurait pas voulu de la malchance de l'enfant albinos. Mais Mamie Adjoua, qui était sa sœur chérie, l'a pris, l'a caché. Quand j'ai accouché, on m'a menti. On a dit à Houphouët que l'enfant était mort. (229)

In a challenge to the broader power structures at work in Yamoussoukro, the accession of the albino to a position of agency represents a reversal of power relations, albeit in an almost fantastical manner.

The Albino Body as a Space of Resistance

Milo's sense of identity – as well as the way in which others see him – is intimately associated with his physical experience of albinism. David Le Breton suggests that:

> A travers sa corporéité, l'homme fait au monde la mesure de son expérience. Il le transforme en un tissu familier et cohérent, disponible à son action et perméable à son expérience. Emetteur ou récepteur, le corps produit continuellement du sens, il insère ainsi activement l'homme à l'intérieur d'un espace social et culturel donné.[26]

Milo's behaviour confirms Le Breton's notion of 'lived' bodily experience, for he both expresses himself and experiences the world through his own body and the bodies of other people. Milo describes his sexual encounters with women as a way of *being*, 'ma façon d'être dans l'une d'elles, dans cet autre monde' (*Mémoire*, 15). The bodies of the women he associates with become an extension of his world, a space of self-discovery. The suggestion is that this experience is mutual as Milo also relates the ways in which other people experience his hidden humanity through intimate encounters with his body. Describing his relationship with his wife Mireille, he comments: 'Chaque fois que nous faisions l'amour, elle sentait de l'humain en moi' (16). It becomes clear that Milo's assertion of his sexuality is one aspect of this two-way process of self-discovery. He describes how difficult it is to forget the body of someone he has loved: 'Rama, la mémoire d'un corps que l'on a aimé est très difficile à effacer' (105). For Milo, so closely bound up is the human body with experience that this memory is almost impossible to erase. The title of Sassine's novel, *Mémoire d'une peau*, is significant then, for it refers to the close association between meaning and the body, or more specifically the skin, for the protagonist of the novel. The title can be interpreted in several ways. Most pertinently for the black African

---

26   David Le Breton, *La Sociologie du corps* (Paris: Presses Universitaires de France, 1992), 4.

with albinism, the memory is of a black skin which defines the individual inclusively in relation to those around him, instead of setting him apart.

Another interpretation of the title is as a reference to the intrinsic memory of skin which retains the marks imposed upon it as a *mémoire* of its experiences. The notion that the albino body is a physical and metaphorical palimpsest, a surface which is inscribed by markings and shaped by the meanings imposed on it, is returned to repeatedly in the novels. The explicit marking of the body discussed in Chapter 3 highlights the ways in which all bodies are socially constructed, bearing as they do inscriptions of gender, race and class. This inscription implies that identities can therefore be constructed through the marking of the body by such processes as scarification, tattooing or the shaping of teeth. However, the body becomes marked in other ways too. Milo refers on several occasions to the scars and scratches on his skin, describing for example the results of a sexual encounter with Rama:

> On s'est fait très mal cette nuit qui n'arrête pas de s'étirer dans ma tête. J'ai gardé des jours les traces de tes ongles sur mon dos, tes morsures sur mes bras, comme des déclarations écrites, le tatouage de nos promesses, ma médaille d'ancien combattant de l'amour. (105)

These marks record his experiences and physical encounters, and while the wrinkles on his face signal his advancing age, they also serve as a record of the suffering he has endured: 'Les plis, les rides de mon visage s'approfondissent, comme des sillons. Je sais que chaque ligne est la conséquence d'une lâcheté, d'une trahison, d'une peur, d'une quête' (8).

The need to complete the albino body and to account for what is perceived to be absent has already been signalled in this study as a fundamental concern of all fictional writing about albinism. Sassine's *Mémoire d'une peau* is no different in suggesting that the discomfort felt at the inability to read into albino skin is compensated for by the inscription of meaning onto it. Connor proposes that, 'in marking the skin, part of the point is to set the skin at naught, to treat it, not as the outward part of the living being, but as an object'.²⁷ Milo's albino skin is described in precisely these terms, inviting inscription like a blank sheet of paper. Working on her typewriter writing a letter to Milo, Rama imagines that she is writing on his body: 'Je tape comme une folle sur la machine comme si c'était ton corps que j'avais sous les doigts' (174). The image of Rama typing on Milo's skin reminds us of the fact that Sassine, Destremau and Grainville are writing on the albino body in a similar way, imposing meaning onto it as Rama leaves scratches on Milo's body which he later reads as a record of their sexual encounters.

Rama's reflections, as well as Milo's references to the marks on his body, recall the notion explored earlier in this study that the albino body is subversive precisely because of the paleness of its skin, which displays the slightest mark made on it for all to see. In his exploration of skin, Connor describes the marks inscribed on the body as the 'order of identity'.²⁸ He argues that 'the order of marks is the order of immediate resemblance, in which everything can be the image of everything else, because everything can both make its mark and be made to bear the mark of everything else'.²⁹ Surveying the inscription of skin, Connor asks what makes the marking of skin different from marking paper. Marked skin, he concludes, means never being able or willing to forget. Certainly, the marking of the albino body serves as a record of that body's experiences and unlike black skin, which Martin suggests was long believed to conceal the marks inflicted on it, albino skin exhibits them.³⁰

The assertion that the body can be written upon implies that it can also be read and Milo mentions this possibility, describing his memories of encounters with others as 'ma mémoire de centaines de corps lus...' (130). Here, the text implies that to 'read' the body, it must be physically experienced, whether intimately or otherwise. In *The Craft of Writing*, William Sloane comments that fiction must be experienced in the same way:

27   Ibid., 82.
28   Ibid., 86.
29   Idem.
30   See Martin, *The White African American Body*, 119.

'[F]iction is as much of a reality as any other experience that the reader undertakes. Call it vicarious if you like, but the reader is not a spectator, he is a participant.'[31] Indeed, it is difficult to read *Mémoire d'une peau* without being drawn into Milo's world and becoming an accomplice to his crimes, as the protagonist invites the reader to participate in his experiences by sharing his perspective on the world, confiding his plans, his feelings and his frustrations.

Milo encounters others through their bodies in many different ways, his sexual relationships being the most obvious means by which he associates with other people. However, the physical nature of his encounters is not always sexual. Milo's relationship with his younger children is close, and characterised by his physical contact with them. He describes playing with them, picking them up and kissing them: 'Marie me posa un bisou sur une tempe. Son frère était en train de se brosser les dents. Je pris la petite sur mes genoux et lui demandai son emploi du temps de la journée' (*Mémoire*, 14). This tenderness towards his children contrasts with the antagonistic relationship beween Milo and his wife. To protect his daughter, Milo sends Marie off to play when her mother, in a fit of anger, suggests he tell his daughter that he is having an affair with her school teacher.

Milo's relationship with his wife Mireille is almost devoid of physical contact and instead is conveyed as an aggressive verbal relationship, constituted by insults and a mutual lack of respect. Milo orders Mireille around: 'Vieille carcasse! N'oublie pas de venir me chercher dans vingt minutes' (17). However, Mireille is Milo's equal when it comes to verbal warfare and there is a sense that the couple are equally deserving of each other. Nevertheless, the final lines of *Mémoire d'une peau* suggest that the couple may feel some sentiment towards each other, however dysfunctional their relationship:

---

31 William Sloane, *The Craft of Writing* (New York: W.W. Norton & Co. Ltd, 1979), 40.

> Je retrouvai ma femme en train de pleurer. Putain de vie je n'aime pas voir une femme pleurer.
> – Arrête, sinon je te casse ta vieille carcasse trop longtemps baisée.
> – T'es un enfant de salaud. Mais je t'aime Milo. (179)

Although never elaborated in the novel, Milo's lack of a physical relationship with his wife suggests a lack of power over her, as it is through the physicality of his relationships that Milo gains control over people. Through his sexual relationship with Hadja, Milo gains the power to expose her as a fraud. Similarly, he reveals Madame Andréa's superficial nature by recounting a relationship with her when she was a young woman, describing her as 'l'intouchable, la super-fidèle, l'ultra-moralisatrice' (112). His relationships with Sister Angélique and Mother Michèle are described in similar terms, as well as his relationships with the wives of people in power, including the Mayor. Likewise, Milo holds power over the married women with whom he has sexual relations by threatening to expose the truth to their husbands. Like the murders he commits, these relationships are a means by which Milo can effect revenge. He follows the advice of his adoptive father, Monsieur Charles, who instructs him:

> Toute la ville t'a vu nu? Il faut que tu baises toute la ville. Quiconque te verra à poil, encule-le. Nous sommes pauvres, nous n'avons que ce morceau de chair entre les cuisses... (42)

The power balance only truly shifts in Milo's romantic relationship with Rama. Early in the narrative, he reveals his desire to fall in love: 'Mon Dieu, donnez-moi une grande histoire d'amour, du fort, de l'immortel pour m'aider. Je suis fatigué de n'être que ce que je suis...' (63), returning to the subject in his letter to Christian and Rama at the end of the narrative, when he writes: 'J'étais depuis longtemps fatigué de ma réputation de faiseur de morts et de sentiments' (157).

Milo does not initially find Rama physically attractive. Nevertheless, he is persuaded by the voice in his head to take a risk and make allowances for the fact that, just as Rama is not like other women, he is not like other men:

Milo Kan, il te faut une femme exceptionnelle. Rama, avec cette somme de tout ce que tu n'aimes pas chez une femme, sera peut-être ton unique amour. Toi aussi, tu n'es pas comme les autres hommes. (69)

Rama is the woman with whom Milo falls in love and as a consequence she gains a degree of power over him. Eventually Milo cannot imagine being without Rama and realises that he has fallen in love for the first time in his life. So important is this to Milo that he describes their relationship in terms of its impact on his physical being, on his very existence: 'J'ai besoin de toi pour respirer, manger, dormir. Je ne suis plus quand tu n'es pas là' (97). However, the balance of power is not all in Rama's favour. The discovery of the bodies of others is also presented in *Mémoire d'une peau* as a claiming of these bodies and Milo refers to his and Christian's relationships with Rama as having resulted in a degree of ownership of her body, suggesting that the power reversal is not complete: 'Le corps de Rama, sa vie, ses petits secrets devaient être remis à nu, dépecés [...]. Elle nous avait appartenu' (131).

Thus Milo lives his life and asserts his identity through his body, or rather in relation to his albino skin. Connor argues that '[t]he very wholeness that the skin possesses preserves its capacity to resume and summarize the whole body.'[32] He notes that the skin is not like an organ, or a nail-clipping, for it is not detachable in such a way that the detached part would remain recognizable. Connor goes on to comment that, 'skin has come to mean the body itself; it has become the definite article, the "the" of the body.'[33] Sassine takes this notion yet further, suggesting that for the person with albinism, the skin defines the individual. This is highlighted in Milo's response to a comment made by his wife regarding his attitude towards other people. When Mireille tells him that he must change, he replies, 'Quand je changerai de peau, je changerai' (14). Expressing his unwillingness to change in relation to his skin, Milo closely associates his personality and his way of being with his outward appearance, a correlation that reveals the profound and lasting impact of Milo's albinism on his life.

---

32   Connor, *The Book of Skin*, 29.
33   Idem.

Although Milo's encounters with other people are described in terms of 'readings' of their bodies, it becomes apparent that the inscrutability of his albino body, echoed in the convoluted narrative of *Mémoire d'une peau*, complicates the process whereby others can 'read' his body. The many associations made with albino skin mean that it is (mis)interpreted as being white, different, deviant, diseased, leprous, symbolic of the supernatural powers of the albino, or a marker of disgrace. The additional layers of meaning attached to the albino body in terms of modern myths and stereotypes are further evidence of the tendency to impose meaning upon what is perceived to be the 'blank' and 'lacking' body of the albino. Thus, the albino body emerges as a multiply inscribed body, which is repeatedly written and rewritten, but which contains layers of residual meaning.

In her study of the figure of the albino in contemporary ethnic American literature, TuSmith suggests that there is a degree of inscrutability associated with the figure of the albino:

> In American society, while the 'inscrutable Oriental' has been *the* stereotype for the Chinese and, by extension, for all peoples of Asian ancestry, one can also find the flip side of this popular image. There exists in both canonical European American and contemporary ethnic American literature the stereotype's counterpart: the 'inscrutable albino'.[34]

TuSmith contends that the albino body is perceived to be blank and consequently inscrutable. However, Sassine's *Mémoire d'une peau* contradicts TuSmith's argument, suggesting instead that the inscrutability of the albino body stems from its complexity. Further complicating the process of reading the albino body is Milo's close association of body with identity and his consequent manipulation of any meaning that is eventually attached to his body. Thus, by examining the constitution, destruction and subsequent reconstruction of albino identity and the way in which it is intimately bound up with the albino body, Sassine draws attention to the need to consider albino identity not in terms of what is lacking – as this study has shown to be so often the tendency in the fictional representation of

---

34   TuSmith, 'The Inscrutable Albino', 85.

this figure – but rather in relation to what is specific to the experience of black African people with albinism. Milo celebrates his difference and his exclusion. He turns the web of beliefs surrounding albinism to his benefit and uses his physical difference and the mystery that surrounds his albino body to attract women. Milo's wife finds out about his affair with their daughter's school mistress and for once, she has evidence:

> C'est vrai qu'elle avait des preuves. Pour une fois qu'on m'écrivait. Une longue lettre semblable aux regards des femmes amoureuses dominant leur mari. Elle avait photocopié sa preuve à des dizaines d'exemplaires à l'intention de tous les cocus de la ville et aux parents d'élèves. (15)

However, Milo is not particularly concerned, for he knows that there will always be women who are interested in him. We learn that this event even enhanced his reputation with the local women: 'La pauvre institutrice avait perdu son poste, mais je gagnai d'autres maîtresses "curieuses"' (15).

By representing the figure of the albino in this way, Sassine highlights the need to move beyond polarised positions on identity towards a more flexible and inclusive position. There has been much discussion about the adequacy of identity in recent years and many indicators signal its continued importance as a topos. A number academic works have been devoted to issues of subjectivity and identity, particularly in relation to discourse, power and the body. As the introduction to this study remarks, there is an ongoing concern with identity in current work on gender, sexuality, race, culture and disability studies, and theorists including Pierre Bourdieu, Claude Lévi-Strauss and Paul Ricœur have written explicitly on the subject, rethinking identity in ways that challenge essentialist paradigms.[35] Perhaps most interesting is the research currently being conducted into the *cyborg* and the idea of the virtual self, because new technologies blur and reconfigure identity boundaries by collapsing distinctions between

---

35   Pierre Bourdieu, 'L'identité et la représentation', *Actes de la recherché en sciences sociales*, 35 (1980) 63–72; Claude Lévi-Strauss, *L'Identité* (Paris: Editions Grasset, 1977), Paul Ricoeur, *Oneself as Another* (Chicago: University of Chicago Press, 1992).

self and other.[36] Other theorists, such as Hall, describe identity as, 'an idea which cannot be thought in the old way, but without which certain key questions cannot be thought at all'.[37] As Ian Ang remarks, 'while we may have discarded identity in theory, we cannot do away with cultural identities as real, social and symbolic forces in history and politics'.[38] There seems to be an over-riding sense that our world has become so fragmented, both ideologically and otherwise, that it is impossible to come to any consensus about identity.

Existing theories of identity fail to fully account for the figure of the albino, focusing only on the problematic associations of the whiteness of the albino body. The constructed nature of albino subjectivity by means of opposition has been a central focus of this study, which has addressed in some detail the processes by which the albino subject is constructed from without, whether this is through myth, stereotype or in relation to colonial hierarchies of white over black, or Western over African. The identification of the figure of the albino as profoundly other results in a double marginalisation, firstly in relation to African identity and secondly in a refusal to attribute any positive qualities to albino identity. Fanon refers to the depersonalisation of the colonised subject in *Peau noire, masques blancs*, as he explores that subject's inability to answer the question, 'qui suis-je?', noting that in the Antillean setting, this was made more acute by racial considerations.[39] Obvious parallels can be drawn with the situation of the black African albino.

Blankenberg proposes that it is necessary to move beyond a consideration of the albino purely in terms of the whiteness of the colonisers:

---

36   See for example, Kim Toffoletti, *Cyborgs and Barbie Dolls: Feminism, Popular Culture and the Posthuman Body* (London: I.B. Tauris & Co., 2007).
37   Stuart Hall, 'Who Needs Identity?' in *The Identity Reader* ed. by Paul du Gay, Jessica Evans and Peter Redman (London: Sage, 2000), 15–31.
38   Ian Ang, 'Identity Blues' in Paul Gilroy, Lawrence Grossberg and Angela McRobbie (eds), *Without Guarantees: In Honour of Stuart Hall* (London: Verso, 2000), 1–14 (2).
39   Fanon, *Peau noire, masques blancs*, 30.

> The Albino was White before the White man came. [...] This White Black person has existed for centuries and continues to exist, the fluidity of his/her being pointing to a rupture in the core African identity of race.[40]

Consideration of the figure of the albino purely in terms of race is inadequate, Blankenberg suggests, because this one feature 'creates a question mark between how one chooses to self-identify and how society and community choose to identify you'.[41] In the body of the albino, the divergence between social and cultural identification on the one hand, and race and physicality on the other, necessitates a re-evaluation of thinking that has assumed for so long that these two things are indivisible.

Bhabha's theoretical readings of Fanon also remind us of the importance of unravelling the binary oppositions which firmly position the African as other and as a result, doubly 'other' the black African albino.[42] Reading otherness as an ambivalent space, Bhabha negotiates a position of resistance from the dismantling of colonial power as a unified or homogenous source. He takes much the same approach to individual identity, examining it from several different theoretical standpoints: cultural, psychoanalytic and post-structuralist. In so doing, he reveals identity to be a process and not a 'thing'. This is the way in which Sassine represents the identity of his protagonist. Realising that people view him purely in relation to his outward appearance, Milo manipulates the ways in which others perceive his albinism, meaning that his identity is never fixed or unified, but by contrast it is disjointed and constantly in a process of change. He overtly manipulates his identity, switching between several different ways of being to suit the situation. Grainville's Alpha and Destremau's Samate also, though less overtly, influence the way in which they are perceived by others. All are characters who develop as the narratives progress, coming to a greater understanding of themselves as individuals and of their position in society. However, the progression is not a smooth one. Instead, the novels present the definition of the subjectivity of the albino as a struggle of community, a negotiation between an individual and the others around him.

40 Blankenberg, 'That Rare and Random Tribe', 13.
41 Ibid., 34.
42 See in particular, Bhabha, 'Remembering Fanon', x.

Kwame Anthony Appiah and Henry Louis Gates suggest that the intersections of race, class and gender are 'a provocative site for the articulation and discussion of new theories and discourses of identity'.[43] Although intersections are indeed interesting positions from which to explore identity, this statement does however raise the question, already referred to briefly in Chapter 4, as to why the figure of the albino must insistently be placed on the margin, his body deemed an excess, or something more. As this study has acknowledged, Destremau, Grainville and Sassine insist on the marginality of their albino protagonists. However, in so doing, they reverse the viewpoint and through their protagonists they turn the questioning on what is deemed to be 'normal', and thus reinstate the figure of the albino. Bell hooks notes the potential of this reversal, arguing that 'One of the most significant forms of power held by the weak is the refusal to accept the definition of oneself that is put forward by the powerful.'[44] hooks suggests that choosing marginality is a critical turning point in the construction of a counter-hegemonic identity. The choice to live out marginality impedes the binary of centre and margin because the margin 'refuses its authoritative definition as other'.[45]

'Être albinos'

In *Wirriyamu* and *Mémoire d'une peau*, Sassine focuses not only on the albino protagonists Condélo and Milo, but also posits various ways in which other people might 'be albino'. Discussing Hadja, the apparently devout Muslim, Milo describes how she invites him into her apartment and, closing the door on the outside world, relaxes and reveals her true

---

43   Kwame Anthony Appiah and Henry Louis Gates, *Identities* (Chicago: University of Chicago Press, 1995), xx.
44   See bell hooks, *Feminist Theory: From Margin to Centre* (Boston: South End Press, 1984), 90.
45   Idem.

self: 'Hadja fermait la porte, soufflait sur la bougie, ôtait sa peau – c'est horrible un adulte qui enlève ses masques' (*Mémoire*, 91). The wearing of masks – in both the literal and metaphorical sense – is a way of hiding the identity of a person and establishing another persona. Living behind their masks, Hadja and others like her become temporarily separated from their own identity. The notion of Hadja 'taking off her skin' brings us back to the notion that the Hadja everyone knows in the outside world is a very different person to the woman she is in the privacy of her own home.

The wearing of masks is closely related to the notion of 'being albino' or, as Sassine suggests through his portrayal of Milo's manipulation of identity, being different things for different people. Milo's curious description of Hadja as 'une albinos à sa façon' (92), is more fully understood when the collocation reappears later in the narrative, as by then it has been more fully developed. When Christian asks Milo how many women he has had relationships with, Milo boasts that he has slept with so many women that he has exhausted the list of saints, from A to Z. Reflecting on these relationships, Milo tells Christian what he learned from the women: 'Elles m'expliquaient à leur façon leur monde, plus grand que la terre, leurs faiblesses, leur marginalité, leur curiosité. Des albinos quoi!' (136). Milo discovers that those around him are all albino in their own way. Being albino then, for Sassine, means being associated with another world; one defined by weakness, marginality and curiosity.

Sassine focuses on this theme throughout his fictional work, a preoccupation that critics relate to the writer's métissage. In an interview with Landry Wilfrid Miampika, Sassine described his personal experiences of métissage:

> Je suis métissé. Mon père est arabe. Ma mère est africaine. Je suis même métissé religieusement. J'ai été chrétien. Je suis maintenant musulman. Mon père était chrétien, quand il est mort je suis devenu musulman à cause de ma mère. Et s'est branchée dessus la culture européenne à travers la culture française.[46]

---

46 Landry-Wilfrid Miampika, 'Exil et marginalité: Entretien avec Williams Sassine'. *Africultures*, http://www.africultures.com/php/index.php?nav=article&no=665 [Accessed 14 January 2010].

Sassine's experiences reflect what Patrick Corcoran terms, 'the ambiguities and dualities inherent within the postcolonial perspective'.[47] Born to a Lebanese Christian father and a Guinean Muslim mother, Sassine's life was divided between Guinea and a period in exile, and he combined a literary career with one in teaching. Asked in an interview about different experiences of *métissage*, Henri Lopes remarks:

> Je crois que Williams Sassine a souffert de son métissage. Il n'en parle pas dans son œuvre. Il fait comme si le métis n'existait pas. [...] Peut-être nous aurait-il donné un beau texte littéraire s'il avait traduit cette douleur en mots ?

Racially *métis* figures are indeed notable for their absence in Sassine's fictional work. However, a number of characters who share Sassine's experiences of cultural and religious *métissage* populate his novels. As Chevrier remarks of Sassine's writing:

> Ecrivain de la marginalité, ainsi que nous l'avons défini [...], Williams Sassine fait en effet vivre sous nos yeux un petit monde de marginaux nés, pour une large part, semble-t-il, de sa propre expérience de métis et d'exilé, une double situation à la fois biologique, sociologique et politique qui a laissé en lui des traces indélébiles.[48]

Intriguingly, in *Mémoire d'une peau*, Sassine extends the experience of marginality associated with albinism to Friedrich Nietzsche. In conversation with Rama, Milo describes how Nietzsche became mad when he discovered that he was albino: 'Ton Nietzsche est devenu dingue quand il a compris. Il s'est découvert albinos' (135). As with many aspects of Sassine's fictional work, the comment is left open to interpretation, but it is notable that once again the association is made between albinism and madness. Milo's repeated references to the little voice in his head suggest schizophrenia. Throughout his œuvre Sassine portrays characters with physical disabilities as mentally ill, among them Ondo in *Wirriyamu*, who sits alone in his hut reading his bible, François in *Saint Monsieur Baly*, who describes himself as 'L'homme-

---

47 Patrick Corcoran, *Lopes: Le Pleurer-Rire* (Glasgow: Glasgow Introductory Guides to French Literature, 2002), 7.
48 Chevrier, *Williams Sassine: écrivain de la marginalité*, 19.

pourri-fou-lépreux-maudit' (89), and Condélo who talks incessantly to his dog. However, as Giguet suggests, 'A l'instar du personnage du fou dans l'ensemble de la société et de la littérature africaines, les fous sassiniens sont souvent plus lucides que le commun des hommes, et leurs propos ne sont incohérents que pour ceux qui en restent à une compréhension littérale.'[49] Ondo tells Kabalango, 'J'ai choisi le camp de la folie, parce qu'il est celui de la sagesse et de la tranquillité' (*Wirriyamu*, 77) and Condélo questions the basis for his judgement by others when he tells his dog, 'C'est moi seul qui parle tout le temps; c'est pour ça peut-être qu'ils ont fini par penser que je suis totalement différent d'eux' (*Wirriyamu*, 30). However, the clearest link between Milo and Nietzsche is nihilism: extreme pessimism and a radical scepticism. Beneath a superficial veneer of sociability Milo is characterized by a dearth of emotion and a lack of belief in anything. He has few loyalties and continually returns to his impulse to destroy. Nihilism is most often associated with Nietzsche who argued that its corrosive effects would eventually destroy all moral, religious, and metaphysical convictions, and bring about the greatest crisis in human history.[50] In these terms, Milo's undermining of the values of the society in which he lives becomes portentous.

In *Wirriyamu*, Condélo also attempts to explain what it means to 'be albino'. In simplistic terms which echo Hegel's master-slave dialectic, Condélo explains the position in which he finds himself to his dog Patience, who accompanies him as he flees for his life:

> Supposons que tu ailles chez un chien plus faible que toi. Tu t'installes chez lui et tu lui dis: 'Tous tes biens m'appartiennent parce que je suis plus fort que toi. Et je suis plus fort que toi, donc tu n'es pas un chien'. Si tu veux faire accepter à ton chien sa nouvelle condition d'esclave, tu dois lui faire croire qu'il est, lui aussi, supérieur à d'autres chiens. S'il ne proteste pas, c'est qu'il accepte en même temps la graduation de l'échelle canine que tu viens d'établir, donc qu'il accepte ta supériorité... Ici, c'est un peu la même chose: les Portugais sont les maîtres des Noirs, et eux sont mes maîtres... (*Wirriyamu*, 54)

---

49 Giguet, 'La construction tragique', unpaginated.
50 Friedrich Nietzsche, *The Will to Power as Art*, translated from the German, with Notes and an Analysis by David Farrell Krell (San Francisco: HarperCollins Publishers, 1991), 9–40.

While Condélo explains the hierarchy which defines the doubly-marginal identity of the albino, he also questions the foundation of the behaviour of others towards him and comes to the conclusion that 'Les hommes, ils sont comme ça; ils ont besoin d'avoir chacun leur fou. Parce qu'à côté d'un fou ils se gonflent et remercient le ciel' (*Wirriyamu*, 30). Condélo's is not only a critique of the colonizers, but of the willingness of other Africans to be persuaded to play a role in a hierarchy which ultimately results in his extreme marginalization and exclusion from society. Like Milo, Condélo uncovers bringing into question the motives of others, and brings under scrutiny 'les bêtises des hommes' (54).

Thus, power and resistance operate on many levels in Sassine's *Mémoire d'une peau*, as well as to a lesser extent in the novels of Destremau and Grainville. Sassine in particular uses humour and the layering of meaning to test, stretch or even break down boundaries, and puts at the disposal of his protagonist tools that have the potential to affirm or to subvert cultural norms. In my examination of the strategies for resistance that are developed in Sassine's *Mémoire d'une peau*, the success of these often subtle, yet subversive forms of resistance in undermining or destabilising dominant discourse has become apparent. By critically addressing his situation, Milo is able to expose the fallacies that refuse him acceptance in society and to come to an understanding of the ways in which his experiences have shaped his identity. In this way, Sassine's narrative addresses the association between power, hegemony, resistance and subordination. Milo criticises, laughs at, undermines and openly condemns the actions of those in positions of authority and of people who believe themselves to be superior to him. His is a form of power exercised from the margins, but one which reveals the hypocritical nature of the society in which he lives and the constructed nature of the categories by which he is excluded as a person with albinism.

However, the novels also show that resistance is closely bound up with power in a complex network of relationships, and this in turn has serious implications on the level of individual identity. The novels demonstrate that the identities of all those positioned within a power relationship – whether in relation to grand power structures or on a more personal level – are constituted through interrelation, with the immediate implication being that this moves beyond the accepted boundaries of the politics of identity. For, not only does the identity of the 'resister' shift and become more complex, but so too does the characterisation of his identity itself. The potential of such a politics of interrelation is profound for the albino, an individual excluded from pre-constituted identity categories.

Blankenberg acknowledges that the nature of albino identity is such that it cannot be universalised or collectivised, commenting that 'It is a lonely identity path. What it has taught me is that little boxes don't fit, identities are fluid.'[51] Given the difficulty of defining the albino body, the possibility of constructing a positive identity as 'albino' must take into consideration the multiple meanings imposed onto this figure. Chapter 2 of this study explored the way in which the establishing of a positive albino identity is problematised by the web of beliefs and misconceptions surrounding the condition, considering the varying ways in which Destremau, Grainville and Sassine take these into account in their portrayal of their protagonists. Chapter 3 focused on inclusion and exclusion, and also addressed the issue of identity, albeit from a different perspective, raising questions concerning the relations of inequality and difference as well as discussing the importance and possibility of a sense of belonging for the albino. However, the novels demonstrate that there is much to add to these perspectives on albino identity – and by implication, African identity – for they raise the question as to whether or not it is possible to move beyond the multiple meanings attached to the albino body. This is a question which has been asked in recent critical writing on albinism and which has also been repeatedly raised by people with the condition.

Albino identity is often constituted in representation in terms of binary oppositions which the albino body does not 'fit'. However, the novels of Destremau, Grainville and Sassine explore the possible alternatives to measuring identity in terms of 'blackness' and 'whiteness' and address the possibility of re-locating and celebrating albinism. In so doing, they posit a more reflexive form of identity construction, which suggests that since albino identity is fundamentally enmeshed in power relations, the albino

---

51   Blankenberg, 'That Rare and Random Tribe', 6.

must subvert instituted structures to create a space where he can locate identity and evade the imposition of identity from without. The novels signal a need to go beyond 'traditional' definitions, theories and categories to account for the figure of the albino, implying that the ideal would be a world in which difference is not highlighted, but rather accepted. It is clear that the way in which the figure of the albino is critically approached also needs rethinking. Given the inadequacy of existing theories of race, disability, colour and difference, it appears that there is a need for new conceptual lenses through which to examine this complex figure.

Conclusion

Destremau, Grainville and Sassine's novels suggest that black Africans with albinism are ultimately defined by the corporeal nature of their identity, whether constructed by the individual or imposed from without. A series of common themes present in different combinations and intensities in the four novels echo the preoccupations of all fictional writing about albinism. These include a recognition of the problematic relationship between inner and outer reality (in both bodily terms and in relation to notions of inclusion and exclusion), the challenging of accepted categories and designations, and the consequent problematisation of the relationship between self and other. Bound up with these issues are questions of identity and power.

In Chapter 1, my analysis of textual representations of the protagonists in the novels of Destremau, Grainville and Sassine demonstrated the importance of the relationship between the individual body and the body politic, identity and its embodiment, and between the subject and dominant discourse for an understanding of this figure. This in turn brought to light the insistently negative portrayal of the albino body in fictional writing. The enduring negativity associated with albinism is reinforced by a series of binary oppositions which the novels explored both highlight and contest. Chapters 2 and 3 demonstrated how boundaries and binary oppositions function to exclude the albino, discussing the ways in which myths and stereotypes operate as a means of enforcing these oppositions by firmly positioning people with albinism as other. As a consequence of these constructed means of containing the ambiguous and the threatening, the albino is pushed to the margins, or in the case of Sassine's Milo, positions himself there. Finally, Chapters 4 and 5 posited the marginal situation of the albino as a potentially powerful one, bringing to light important questions about the way in which postcolonial African society is structured.

My discussion has shown that the negativity that continues to surround the figure of the albino in much of contemporary sub-Saharan Africa is intrinsic to fictional writing about albinism. This negativity results in part from the ways in which bodily difference and deviance are represented as integral to the shaping of the identity of the figure of the albino. Attempts to explain the albino body in terms of existing categories – as 'white', 'disabled' or simply 'different' – have resulted in a range of responses to this ambiguous figure, the majority of which are far from positive. The negativity surrounding albinism operates as a form of negation, an attempt to push this figure to the boundaries in a type of exclusion which, the novels demonstrate, functions to reinforce the difference of the albino in order to protect and confirm the normality of the Self.

The need to explain and contain albinism is evidenced in the beliefs and stereotypes that continue to shape perceptions of people with the condition. These attempts to classify and control are reflected in the themes of deviance, marginality and exclusion which are integral to the work of Destremau, Grainville and Sassine. Although *Nègre blanc*, *Le Tyran éternel*, *Wirriyamu* and *Mémoire d'une peau* are very different novels, written from different perspectives, all four portray the fear surrounding the figure of the albino, which often results from an ignorance of albinism and apprehension with regard to the unknown. The writers suggest that integral to this fear is the notion of a potential threat posed by the indecipherable albino body. While this approach could be considered to give a purely negative perspective on albinism, it reflects the reality of living with the condition in contemporary sub-Saharan Africa, where the majority of people with albinism remain marginalised by the attitudes of others. By focusing on such issues, the novels go some way towards highlighting the difficulties faced by people with albinism in their everyday lives.

Destremau, Grainville and Sassine's representations of albinism suggest that the presence of albinism raises many questions about the ways in which we structure the world. In my discussion of the notion of threat and the drawing of boundaries, I addressed the apparent need to define the people with albinism in terms of binaries which the black African albino body at once emphasises and challenges. Choices between black and white result from a continued adherence to the binary oppositions which were reinforced under colonialism, and which continue to hold currency today. In Martin's terms, 'racial difference still remains, blackness and whiteness continuing their incestuous dance'.[1] As I discussed in Chapter 1, the choice

---

1   Martin, *The White African American Body*, 184.

Conclusion

as to whether to define people with albinism as able-bodied or disabled emerges as equally problematic. All four novels demonstrate the ways in which the attitudes of others aggravate the situation of people with albinism, often constituting a more significant disability than the physical limitations resulting from the condition itself.

For black and for white, for colonised and coloniser, for able-bodied and disabled, the novels of Destremau, Grainville and Sassine suggest that the albino body is disturbing because of its troubling similarity to the body of the onlooker. Blankenberg expresses the tension between the black body and the white body in terms of a rupture:

> My grandfather, as black as tar, was ecstatic. The gods had decided to give him a white grandson; almost white, but not quite. As I got older, people would look at me with horror, with fascination, almost perfect but not quite, and, for a minute, their sense of the ways of the world was ruptured. Just by looking.[2]

The rupture described by Blankenberg is one of identity and the established bounded categories that define it. This rupture expresses the profound and problematic associations of the albino body. The albino body becomes powerfully uncanny and threatening to the comfortable binaries of black and white, dominated and dominant.

Sassine's *Wirriyamu* shows that in pre-colonial Africa, the visible physical difference of people with albinism marked them apart, and mythical and mystical associations were attached to the albino body that continue to hold currency today. However, as *Nègre blanc*, *Le Tyran éternel* and *Mémoire d'une peau* demonstrate, the distinctive appearance of people with albinism has also become culturally significant in postcolonial Africa. Although the lack of pigmentation does not make the person with albinism white in racial terms, it means that this figure has been interpreted as a walking embodiment of the dilemma faced by postcolonial societies that have become deeply sensitised to racialised forms of thinking and acting. Bringing about a questioning of the binary oppositions that shape the postcolonial world, fictional representations of the figure of the albino reveal the basic concepts in this discourse to be produced by relations of power.

2   Blankenberg, 'That Rare and Random Tribe', 7.

In Chapter 4 I discussed Bhabha's contention that the lines or spaces of division between binaries are the loci of power. In *The Location of Culture* Bhabha suggests that 'At the edge, in-between the Black body and the White body, there is a tension of meaning and being, or some would say, demand and desire. It is from such tensions [...] that a strategy of subversion emerges.'[3] Discussing Fanon's *Peau noire, masques blancs*, he argues that in the uncertainty of the white-masked black man, and from such ambivalent identification, it is possible to transform cultural confusion into a strategy of political subversion.[4] In Chapter 5 I argued that the same 'tension of meaning and being' is found in the albino body, and that consequently it functions as a site for articulating power. In *Mémoire d'une peau* in particular, Sassine suggests that because the albino body is apparently unconfined by boundaries and consequently resists interpretation, it threatens to become subversive. Recognition of the fear associated with the perceived threat posed by the albino body is manipulated by the protagonist into an assertion of his difference and consequently an – albeit limited – assertion of power.

Although albino identity is often constituted in representation through discursive exclusion, in terms of binary oppositions which the albino body does not 'fit', Destremau, Grainville and Sassine explore the alternatives to simply measuring identity in relation to these binaries and address the possibility of re-locating and celebrating albino identity. In so doing, they posit a more reflexive form of identity construction, suggesting that since albino identity is fundamentally enmeshed in power relations, identity must be established from the margins. The figure of the albino must subvert instituted structures to create a space in which he can locate identity and evade the imposition of identity from without.

Appiah and Gates propose that the intersections of 'race', class and gender are 'a provocative site for the articulation and discussion of new theories and discourses of identity'.[5] Although intersections are indeed

---

3   Bhabha, *The Location of Culture*, 62.
4   Idem.
5   Appiah and Gates, *Identity*, 16.

interesting positions from which to explore the notion of identity, this statement does raise the question as to why the figure of the albino must insistently be placed at the margins. Destremau, Grainville and Sassine insist on the marginal position of their albino protagonists, but their novels are distinct from many other fictional representations of albinism in suggesting that the margins are not a negative space, but instead a space of possibility. Bell hooks sees the potential in this approach, contending that, 'One of the most significant forms of power held by the weak is the refusal to accept the definition of oneself that is put forward by the powerful.'[6] hooks suggests that choosing marginality is a critical turning point in the construction of a counter-hegemonic identity. The choice to live out marginality impedes the binary of centre and margin because the margin refuses its authoritative definition as other. Rather than positing the margins as a purely negative space, Destremau, Grainville and Sassine suggest that the margin or space 'in-between' is a place from which identity can be performed and contested.

Despite the empowering potential of positioning the figure of the albino in the margins, it is important to acknowledge the impact of insistently negative representations of albinism on people with the condition. In the light of such negative representations, people with albinism have been faced with a choice: either to accept and celebrate their albino identity or to argue that albinism is not all-defining. The first position, taken by Blankenberg, confirms identification as a person with albinism as a valid decision, and one that celebrates difference and signals belonging to a select group by way of deviation from the black African 'norm'.[7] Blankenberg asserts that the physical difference of people with albinism is a defining feature, a position shared by Grainville, who represents the meeting between Alpha and Salif as a significant moment in *Le Tyran éternel*. By asserting a particular and distinct albino identity, Salif convinces Alpha that accepting difference and celebrating a previously marginal identity is possible. However, a second position is sometimes taken, as demonstrated

---

6   See hooks, 'marginality as site of resistance', 90.
7   Blankenberg, 'That Rare and Random Tribe', 7.

by Sassine's portrayal of Milo's manipulation of his labelling as 'albino'. This classification typifies the tendency of representation to situate the individual's being in a causal relationship with his albinism, effectively removing the person from the equation.

The presence of the figure of the albino in sub-Saharan Africa, and in fictional representations of colonial and postcolonial Africa, not only raises questions about albino identity, but also brings into question what precisely constitutes African identity. Grainville's Sylvanus comments, 'l'Albinos [...] c'est notre visage encore, le plus provocant, le plus bouleversant, voilà!' (*Tyran*, 84), suggesting that the presence of the albino invites a self-reflexive consideration of what it means to be African. Appiah remarks that in the pre-colonial era, with limited contact between Africa and the West, there was no 'African identity' as such, suggesting that the feeling of a common unity was forced upon African people by the colonial conquest which brought larger political units, common languages and resulted in the breakdown of many traditional institutions.[8] Appiah argues that the negative experiences of slavery and colonialism brought Africa as a unity into being. Africans from many different regions were taken as slaves to the Americas where cultural differences were rooted out by force or slowly faded with time. The common denominator was the increasingly mythologised continent of origin. The concept of 'Africa' grew stronger and from these negative experiences developed counter forces which led to a positive idea of African unity. Pan-Africanism, Négritude and black pride were all based around a common black identity in the face of the hegemony and domination of the colonisers. In the postcolonial world, the figure of the albino stands between two worlds, a Western world and an African one, because he is positioned as the other of African identity (not being black) and the other in Western discourse (not being white). The chromatic ambivalence of the albino body challenges notions of black African universality on which movements such as Négritude were founded, leading Blankenberg to suggest that the figure of the albino necessitates a revisioning of what it means to be African:

8   Appiah, *In My Father's House*, 174.

Conclusion

> In theory [...] the Albino leads the way to the fracturing of the concept of race. In practice, in life (and especially in death), the Albino ruptures an essential sense of African identity, forces a questioning of an African epistemology and paves a new course for a contemporary recognition of an African self.[9]

The albinism of the protagonists at the heart of Destremau, Grainville and Sassine's novels functions as a reminder of the pre-colonial past, which still influences the everyday lives of many people in Africa. At the same time, the novels signal the need for a move towards the inclusion of previously marginalised figures. Sassine's novels in particular draw attention to a change in the way in which notions of the individual and society have evolved. In both *Wirriyamu* and *Mémoire d'une peau*, Sassine focuses on the emergence of the individual in societies which have always put the emphasis on the community. However, in so doing, he also argues for a return to the communal values of African societies. As Chevrier notes:

> Il est clair que la préférence du romancier va à des héros solitaires qui incarnent le drame d'une société postcoloniale dans la mesure où ils vivent simultanément la rupture avec l'univers traditionnel du passé et la tentative d'ouverture à la modernité.[10]

Sassine's novels suggest that a society is defined by the way in which it treats its marginal members. The flaws in the societies in which both Condélo and Milo live are revealed and critiqued by Sassine. He exposes the exploitation of Condélo in the colonial society of *Wirriyamu*, demonstrating the power of myth and the tendency to use the figure of the albino as a scapegoat. By contrast, colour-based prejudice is predominant in the postcolonial setting of *Mémoire d'une peau*. Sassine suggests that only by incorporating marginal individuals into society is it possible to challenge absolutism and dispute the continued reliance on Manichean binaries, many of which were put in place under colonialism. The inclusion of people with albinism opens up positive implications for the reconsideration of African identity, for this figure demands a re-examination of what constitutes the postcolonial African self, a self not simply defined in terms dictated by the colonisers.

9   Blankenberg, 'That Rare and Random Tribe', 8.
10 Chevrier, *Williams Sassine*, 6.

Discussion of the concept of identity raises the question as to whether or not there was ever a time when cohesive identity formations existed, or whether such claims were purely constructed, as under colonialism. Identity has long been understood as a means of constructing legitimating boundaries, and in turn, cultural power. The novels explored here tend to portray the figure of the albino in relation to binary oppositions and bounded categories, failing to embrace a more open and inclusive way of viewing the world. However, this study has shown that the identity of the albino is never unitary, never stable, nor entirely coherent, and that herein lie possibilities, not only on the level of individual identity, but also on a grander scale for contesting accepted ideologies. As Chapter 5 of this study established, Sassine's *Mémoire d'une peau* plays on the very fact that individuals possess multiple identities and that the self is marked by the intersection of multiple subject positions, any of which may take priority in a given situation. This instability of identity (and consequently identification) is central to Milo's assertion of individuality and his challenging of power structures within the society in which he lives. Although the novels signal a need to go beyond conventional definitions, theories and categories to account for the figure of the albino, only Sassine's *Wirriyamu* proposes a world in which difference is accepted. Condélo dreams of a utopian world, 'où il n'y a ni Noirs, ni Blancs, ni albinos' (120).

While some theorists argue that an individual assumes different identities at different times and that identity is a matter of 'becoming' as well as 'being', others consider that it is time to move beyond identity. Cooper contends that identity 'tends to mean too much, too little or nothing at all'.[11] For Cooper, the notion that identities are constructed, fluid and multiple leaves us without a rationale for talking about identities, and leaves the critic ill-equipped to examine the essentialist claims of contemporary identity politics. The limits of traditional identity categories such as those of race, gender, class, nationality and sex, have consistently dismissed or excluded various marginalised groups from their theoretical and practical apparatuses. Indeed, people with albinism are excluded from many of

---

11   Cooper, *Colonialism in Question*, 59.

Conclusion

these categories on the basis of physical, sexual and/or mental inadequacy, although gender and nationality offer alternative points of identification for individuals who would otherwise be excluded. Sassine in particular suggests that there is a need to explore alternatives and to move beyond notions of identity that perpetuate colonising discourses of difference towards those that recognise the uniqueness of individuals.

Just as it has been difficult to account for the figure of the albino in terms of existing categories, it appears that no one critical perspective is adequate to fully account for representations of the figure of the albino. Given the inadequacy of existing theories of race, ability and disability, colour, normality and difference, it seems necessary to move beyond these long-established categories in order to fully account for albinism. Reflecting on her discussion of albino identity, Blankenberg comments that there is a need for new theoretical lenses through which to examine the figure of the black African albino: 'It has taught me that the tools that I use to explore others and myself must be as varied as the selves they describe.'[12] In *Enduring Negativity*, the use of postcolonial theory has permitted a comparative and interdisciplinary approach to the study of representations of albinism. This has enabled me to consider the novels studied in relation to socio-cultural understandings of albinism. I have also been able to draw on recent research in fields as diverse as anthropology, genetics, geography and sociology, which has provided as broad an understanding of the reality of living with albinism as possible. The focus on the four selected novels has permitted a close reading of each narrative, shedding new critical light on these under-studied writers. However, the need to focus and contain the study has meant that it has not been possible to follow up certain points of interest beyond a brief mention. It has been impossible to convey the scale and nature of the social and health issues relating to albinism in this study. Most pressing is the continued work to resolve the practical issues faced by people with albinism in sub-Saharan Africa in their everyday lives, providing them with access to education and employment. This in turn involves – and perhaps depends on – the monumental task of changing

---

12 Blankenberg, 'That Rare and Random Tribe', 6.

attitudes, some of which have existed for centuries, have been aggravated by the impact of colonialism, and which continue to evolve today into a web of modern myths. The focus on sub-Saharan Africa has meant that I have not been able to compare the experiences of people with albinism from other cultures with those of the black African albino. Equally, because of the focus of the novels, and consequently the study, on male black African albino protagonists, I have not been able to address the specific problems encountered by black African women with albinism. The different experiences of people with albinism from different ethnic groups in the West, and representations of people with albinism in apartheid South Africa were both beyond the scope of this study, but I am currently exploring these elsewhere. The number of characters with albinism appearing in films in recent years means that a study of filmic representations and particularly of the stereotypical albino villain would have much to add to current understandings of perceptions of this figure.[13] As I have indicated in this study, characters with albinism appear in oral literature and folk tales, and a comparative study of representations of albinism in oral literature and the contemporary African novel would be a way of tracing changing attitudes towards people with albinism.[14] There is also significant interest to be gained from further studies of the fictional representation of albinism, particularly in light of the broader relevance of the experiences of people with albinism to those of people with other visible disabilities.

Given the relative lack of critical attention to the figure of the albino, the aim here has been to draw attention to and explore the over-ridingly negative portrayal of albinism in order to bring about a new understanding of the potential of the figure of the albino in representation. Critical analyses of the portrayal of albinism have an important role to play in the changing of attitudes, for fictional representation has the potential to

---

13 Val Reese has compiled a comprehensive list of over seventy films with albino characters. See <http://www.skinema.com> [Accessed 28 May 2009].

14 Françoise Parent Ugochukwu has researched the meaning of colour in folk tales, but has not looked specifically at albinism. See Françoise Parent Ugochukwu, 'The Devil's Colours: A Comparative Study of French and Nigerian Folktales', *Oral Tradition*, 21.2 (2007), 1–18.

influence attitudes towards people with albinism, whether positively or negatively. One of the key insights I hope to have given into the experiences of people with albinism is that they are plural, fluid and changing. Awareness of the plurality of experiences of people with the condition is essential if the stereotypes of albinism are to be combated. It has also become clear that the ambiguities associated with the figure of the albino – a figure that embodies and challenges notions of centre and margin, self and other, to which I have tried to give expression in this study – must be taken account of. However, the nature of the albino, who is in Bhabha's terms 'almost the same, but not white',[15] means that attempts to represent this figure raise as many questions as attempts to critique those representations.

15   Bhabha, *The Location of Culture*, 89.

APPENDIX

Fictional Works Featuring Albino Characters

Characters in these novels and short stories are albino, or are attributed albinic features and qualities.

Agualusa, José Eduardo, *The Book of Chameleons* (London: Arcadia Books, 2006)
Bester, Alfred, *The Stars My Destination* (London: Vintage, 1996)
Biemiller, Carl L., *The Albino Blue* (New York: Doubleday, 1998)
Brown, Dan, *The Da Vinci Code* (London: Corgi, 2004)
Carney, Danile, *The Whispering Death* (Bath: Chivers Press Ltd, 1987)
Cauley, Jack E., *Albino Joe* (London: Vantage, 1995)
Chabin, Laurent, *Serdarin des étoiles* (Saint-Laurent: Tisseyre, 1998)
Cheney-Coker, Syl, *The Last Harmattan of Alusine Dunbar: A Novel of Magical Vision* (London: Heinemann, 1990)
Coulibaly, Niama, *Mort d'un albinos* (Bamako: Le Figuier, 1996).
Danticat, Edwidge, *Breath, Eyes, Memory* (New York: Random House, 1998)
Des Roches, Rogers, *Les Idées noires d'Amélie Blanche* (Montreal: Québec Amérique Jeunesse, 2003)
Destremau, Didier, *Nègre blanc* (Paris: Editions Hatier International, 2002)
Dunn, Katherine, *Geek Love* (New York: Warner, 2002)
Farnes, Catherine, *Snow* (Greenville: Bob Jones University Press, 1999)
Fardoulis-Legrange, Michel, *Les Caryatides et l'albinos* (Paris: Jose Corti, 2002)
Fitch, Janet, *White Oleander* (New York: Little, Brown and Company, 1999)
Foster, David, *Moonlite* (New York: Penguin USA, 1988)
Frazier, Charles, *Cold Mountain* (Boston: Atlantic Press, 1997)
Grainville, Patrick, *Le Tyran éternel* (Paris: Editions du Seuil, 1998)
Hand, Elizabeth, *Winterlong* (New York: Eos, 1997)
Hanson, Ben J., *Takadini* (Harare: Fidalyn, 1997)
Harvill, Ken, *Kill Whitey* (Los Angeles: Uglytown Productions, 2005)
Hay, Sheridan, *The Secret of Lost Things* (London: Doubleday, 2007)
Hemingway, Amanda, *The Greenstone Grail* (New York: Voyager, 2004)
———, *The Sword of Straw* (New York: DelRay, 2006)
Hill, Ernestine, *Johnnie Wisecap* (Charlotte: Walkabout, 1998)

Hong Kingston, Maxine, *The Woman Warrior: Memoirs of a Girlhood Among Ghosts* (London: Vintage, 1989)
Kiernan, Caitlín, *Threshold* (New York: Onyx Books, 2001)
———, *In the Garden of Poisonous Flowers* (Burton, Michigan: Subterranean Press, 2002)
———, *Alabaster* (Burton, Michigan: Subterranean Press, 2006)
Kinsella, W.P., *The Iowa Baseball Confederacy: A Novel* (New York: Houghton Mifflin, 1986)
Lawrence, Iain, *Ghost Boy* (New York: Laure Leaf, 2002)
Makhélé, Caya, *Les travaux d'Ariane suivi de Destins et de Quelque part en ce monde* (Paris: Asphalte/Acoria, 2009)
Markandaya, Kamala, *Nectar in a Sieve* (Colchester: Signet, 2002)
Martin, Guy, *L'Albinos ou la légende du dieu Atchafalaya* (Paris: Editions Seuil, 2000)
Maynard, Meredith, *Blue True Dream of Sky* (New York: Polestar, 2000)
McCarthy, Cormac, *Blood Meridian or the Evening Redness in the West* (London: Vintage, 1992)
McGarry Morris, Mary, *Songs in Ordinary Times* (New York: Penguin USA, 1996)
Miller, Alyce, *Color Struck* (New York: Norton & Company, 1995)
Min, Katherine, *Secondhand World* (New York: Knopf, 2006)
Momaday, Scott, *House Made of Dawn* (New York: Harper Perennial, 1999)
Moorcock, Michael, *The Revenge of the Rose: A Tale of the Albino Prince in his Years of Wandering* (Los Angeles: Grafton, 1991)
———, *The Dreamthief's Daughter: A Tale of the Albino* (New York: Warner, 2002)
———, *The White Wolf's Son: The Albino in the Middle March* (New York: Warner, 2005)
Muir, Richard, *The Miniature Man* (New York: St Martin's Press, 1987)
Niven, Larry, *The Burning City* (New York: Pocket Books, 2001)
Nyonda, Vincent de Paul, *La Mort de Guykafi, suivi de deux albinos à la M'Passa* (Paris: L'Harmattan, 1981).
Okri, Ben, *The Famished Road* (London: Vintage, 1992)
Peck, Dale, *Now It's Time to Say Goodbye* (New York: Quill, 1999)
Pinguilly, Yves, *Manèges dans le désert* (Paris: Editions Nathan, 2001)
Platt, Randall Beth, *The Likes of Me* (New York: Laure Leaf, 2001)
Prior, Lily, *Nectar* (New York: Ecco, 2003)
Pynchon, Thomas, '*V*' (New York: Harper Perennial, 1999)
Roy, Namba, *Black Albino* (Harlow: Longman, 1961)
Sassine, Williams, *Wirriyamu* (Paris: Editions Présence Africaine, 1976)
———, *Mémoire d'une peau* (Paris: Editions Présence Africaine, 1998)

Fictional Works Featuring Albino Characters

Segalen, Dominique, *Albus* (Paris: Broché, 2006)
Skene, Anthony, *Monsieur Zenith, The Albino* (London: Savoy, 1935)
Smith, Dale, *The Albino's Dancer* (London: Telos Publishing, 2006)
Soyinka, Wole, *The Interpreters* (London: Fontana, 1986)
Stuefloten, D., *The Wilderness* (Tallahassee: FC2, 2000)
Watts, Leander, *Wild Ride to Heaven* (New York: Houghton Mifflin, 2003)
Wells, H.G., *The Invisible Man* (London: Signet, 2002)
Wideman, John Edgar, *Sent for You Yesterday* (Washington: Houghton Mifflin, 1998)

Bibliography

Primary texts

Destremau, Didier, *Nègre blanc* (Paris: Hatier International, 2002).
Grainville, Patrick, *Le Tyran éternel* (Paris: Editions du Seuil, 1998).
Sassine, Williams, *Mémoire d'une peau* (Paris: Présence Africaine, 1998).
Sassine, Williams, *Wirriyamu* (Paris: Présence Africaine, 1976).

Secondary sources

Abadi, R.V. and E. Pascal, 'The Recognition and Management of Albinism', *Opthalmic Physiol Opt*, 9 (1989), 3–15.
Adebayo, Aduke Grace, 'The Social Function of the African Novel', *Neohelicon*, 16.2 (1989), 73–88.
Aguirre, Manuel, Roberta Quance and Philip Sutton, *Margins and Thresholds: An Enquiry into the Concept of Liminality in Text Studies* (Madrid: Gateway Press, 2000).
Alexandre, Pierre, 'Un conte bulu de Sangmelina: la jeune albinos et le pygmée', *Journal des Africainistes*, 32 (1963), 243–54.
Allen, Theodore, *The Invention of the White Race* (London: Verso, 1994).
Alwan, A. and B. Modell, 'Recommendations for Introducing Genetic Services in Developing Countries', *Nature Reviews Genetics*, 4 (2003), 61–8.
Amondji, Marcel, *Félix Houphouët-Boigny et la Côte d'Ivoire: l'envers d'une légende* (Paris: Karthala, 1985).
Amselle, Jean-Loup and M'Boloko Elikia, *Au coeur de l'ethnie: ethnie, tribalisme et Etat en Afrique* (Paris: La Découverte, 1999).
Amuta, Chidi, *The Theory of African Literature* (London: Institute for African Alternatives, 1989).

Angus, Ian, *A Border Within: National Identity, Cultural Plurality and Wilderness* (Montreal: McGill Queens University Press, 1997).
Anzaldúa, Gloria, *Borderlands/La Frontera: The New Mestiza* (San Francisco: Aunt Lute, 1987).
Anzieu, Didier, *Le Moi-peau* (Paris: Dunod, 1990).
——, *Une peau pour les pensées* (Paris: Apsygée, 1995).
Appiah, Kwame Anthony, *In My Father's House: Africa in the Philosophy of Culture* (Oxford: Oxford University Press, 1992).
——, and Henry Louis Gates, Jr., *Identities* (London: University of Chicago Press, 1995).
Aquaron, Robert, 'Regards sur les albinos africains' in *L'Autre et nous*, ed. by P. Blanchard, S. Blanchain, N. Bancel, G. Boetsch and H. Gerbeau (Paris: Syros et Achac, 1995), pp. 89–93.
——, 'Oculocutaneous Albinism in Cameroon: A Fifteen Year Follow Up Study', *Ophthalmic Paediatrics Genet*, 11 (1990), 255–63.
Aquaron, Robert, Médard Djatou and Luc Kamdem, 'Aspects socioculturels des albinos en Afrique Noire: des mutilations et crimes rituels perpétrés en Afrique de l'est (Burundi et Tanzanie)', *Tropical Medicine*, 69.5 (2009), 449–53.
Aspel, Elizabeth, Barbara Christian and Helene Moglen, eds, *Female Subjects in Black and White: Race, Psychoanalysis, Feminism* (London: University of California Press, 1997).
Awkward, Michael, *Negotiating Difference: Race, Gender and the Politics of Positionality* (London: Chicago University Press, 1995).
Azoulay, Gibel, *Black, Jewish & Interracial* (Durham: Duke University Press, 1997).
Babb, Valerie, *Whiteness Visible: The Meaning of Whiteness in American Literature and Culture* (New York: New York University Press, 1998).
Back, Les, and John Solomos, *Theories of Race and Racism: A Reader* (London: Routledge, 1999).
Bah, Mahmoud, *Construire la Guinée: Après Sékou Touré* (Paris: L'Harmattan, 1990).
Baker, Charlotte, 'Etre albinos: The Trope of Albinism in Williams Sassine's *Wirriyamu* and *Mémoire d'une peau*', *International Journal of Francophone Studies* 13.1 (2010) 9–22.
——, ed., *Expressions of the Body: Representations in African Text and Image* (Oxford: Peter Lang, 2009).
Baker, Charlotte, and Médard Djatou, 'Literary and Anthropological Perspectives on the Black African Albino' in *Crossing Places: New Research in African Studies*, ed. by Charlotte Baker and Zoë Norridge (Newcastle: Cambridge Scholars Publishing, 2007), pp. 63–75.

Baker, Charlotte, Patricia Lund, Julie Taylor and Richard Nyathi, 'The Myths Surrounding People with Albinism in Southern Africa', *Journal of African Cultural Studies* 22.2 (2010).
Bakhurst, David, and Christine Sypnowich, *The Social Self: Inquiries in Social Construction* (London: Sage, 1995).
Bakhtin, Mikhail, *Rabelais and his World* (Bloomington: Indiana University Press, 1984).
Bammer, Angelika, ed., *Displacements–Cultural Identities in Question* (Bloomington: Indiana University Press, 1994).
Banks, Kathryn and Joseph Harris, eds, *Exposure: Revealing Bodies, Unveiling Representations* (Oxford: Peter Lang, 2004).
Banton, M., *Discrimination* (Milton Keynes: Open University Press, 1994).
Bardolph, Jacqueline, ed., *Littérature et maladie en Afrique* (Paris: L'Harmattan, 1994).
Barkow, J.H., 'The Distance Between Genes and Culture', *Journal of Anthropological Research*, 42.3 (1986), 373–85.
Bastide, Roger, *La Notion de personne en Afrique noire* (Paris: CNRS, 1973).
Bay, Mia, *The White Image in the Black Mind* (Oxford: Oxford University Press, 2000).
Belal, Karim, and Philippe Blanchot, 'Salif Keita: Un homme blanc au sang noir', *Afrique Magazine*, 133 (1996), 38–41.
Benthien, Claudia, *Skin: On the Cultural Border between Self and the World* (New York: Columbia University Press, 2002).
——, 'The Whiteness Underneath the Nigger: Albinism and Blackness in Wideman's *Sent for you Yesterday*', *Utah Foreign Language Review*, 56 (1997), 3–13.
Berger, Maurice, *White Lies: Race and the Myths of Whiteness* (New York: Farrar, Strauss and Giroux, 1999).
Bernabé, Jean, Patrick Chamoiseau and Raphaël Confiant, *Eloge de la créolité* (Paris: Gallimard, 1993).
Bestman, Martin T., *Le Jeu des masques: essai sur le roman africain* (Paris: Nouvelle Optique, 1980).
Bhabha, Homi K., *The Location of Culture* (London and New York: Routledge, 1994).
——, 'Remembering Fanon', Foreword to Fanon, *Black Skin, White Masks* (London: Pluto Press, 1986).
Billington, Rosamund, Jenny Hockey and Sheelagh Strawbridge, *Exploring Self and Society* (Basingstoke: Palgrave, 1998).
Biswas, S., and I. Lloyd, 'Oculocutaneous Albinism', *Archives of Disease in Childhood*, 80 (1999), 565–9.

Blankenberg, Ngaire, 'That Rare and Random Tribe: Albino Identity in South Africa', *Critical Arts*, 14.2 (2000), 6–48.
Boehmer, Elleke, *Empire, the National, and the Postcolonial: Resistance in Interaction* (Oxford: Oxford University Press, 2002).
Bogdan, Robert, *Freak Show: Presenting Human Oddities for Amusement and Profit* (Chicago: University of Chicago Press, 1988).
Boime, Albert, *The Art of Exclusion: Representing Blacks in the Nineteenth Century* (Washington: Smithsonian Institution Press, 1990).
Bokiba, André-Patient, *Ecriture et identité dans la littérature africaine* (Paris: L'Harmattan, 1998).
Boni, Tanella, 'L'Ecrivain et le pouvoir', *Notre Librarie*, 98 (1989), 82–91.
Bonnet, Alastair, *White Identities: Historical and International Perspectives* (Harlow: Prentice Hall, 2000).
Borel, France, *Le Vêtement incarné* (Paris: Calmann-Lévy, 1992).
Boskin, Joseph, *Rebellious Laughter: People's Humor in American Culture* (New York: Syracuse University Press, 1997).
Bourdieu, Pierre, 'L'Identité et la représentation', *Actes de la recherche en sciences sociales*, 35 (1980), 63–72.
Bourdillon, M., *The Shona Peoples* (Gweru, Zimbabwe: Mambo Press, 1987).
Boyer, Monique, *Métisse* (Paris: L'Harmattan, 1992).
Brah, Avtar, Mary J. Hickman and Mairtin Mac an Ghail, eds, *Thinking Identities: Ethnicity Racism and Culture* (Basingstoke: Macmillan, 1999).
Butler, Judith, *Bodies That Matter: On the Discursive Limits of Sex* (London: Routledge, 1993).
Caplan, Jane, *Written on the Body* (London: Reaktion, 2002).
Carnegie, Charles V., 'The Dundus and the Nation' *Cultural Anthropology* 11.4 (1996) 470–509.
——, *Postnationalism Prefigured* (New Brunswick: Rutgers University Press, 2002).
Cassuto, Leonard, *The Inhuman Race: The Racial Grotesque in American Literature and Culture* (New York: Columbia University Press, 1997).
Castells, Manuel, *The Power of Identity* (London: Blackwell, 1997).
Cavell, Marcia, *Becoming a Subject: Reflections in Philosophy and Psychoanalysis* (Oxford: Clarendon Press, 2006).
Chamoiseau, Patrick, *Chronique des sept misères* (Paris: Gallimard, 1986).
Chelala, Ninou and Pascale Jeambrun, *L'albinos en Afrique: La blancheur noire énigmatique* (Paris: Broché, 2007).
Cherki, Alice, *Frantz Fanon: A Portrait* (Ithaca and London: Cornell University Press, 2006).
Chevrier, Jacques, *Le Lecteur d'Afriques* (Paris: Honoré Champion, 2005).
——, *La Littérature nègre* (Paris: Armand Colin, 1999).

Bibliography

——, 'Malades et infirmes dans l'œuvre romanesque de Williams Sassine' in *Littérature et maladie dans la littérature africaine* ed. by Jacqueline Bardolph (Paris: L'Harmattan, 1994) pp. 173–87.

——, 'La Marginalité, figure du postcolonialisme dans l'œuvre romanesque de Williams Sassine' in *Littératures postcoloniales et francophonie* ed. by Jean Bessière and Jean-Marc Moura (Paris: Champion, 1999), pp. 131–9.

——, 'De la solitude à la solidarité dans l'œuvre romanesque de Williams Sassine', *Notre Librairie*, 128 (1996), 126–32.

——, 'Le Thème de l'exclusion et de la marginalité dans l'œuvre de Williams Sassine' in *Carrefour de cultures* ed. by Régis Antoine (Tubingen, 1993) pp. 431–8.

——, 'Williams Sassine: Des mathématiques à la littérature', *Notre Librairie*, 88–9 (1987), 110–18.

——, *Williams Sassine: écrivain de la marginalité* (Toronto: Editions du Gref, 1995)

Chinweizu, Unwuchekwa Jemi J., and Ihechukwu Madubuike, *Toward the Decolonization of African Literature* (Enugu: Fourth Dimension Publishers, 1980).

Clasen, Bettina, 'Être albinos en Afrique', *Images*, 41 (1999), 11–15.

Conboy, Katie, Nadia Medina and Sarah Stanbury, eds, *Writing on the Body: Female Embodiment and Feminist Theory* (New York: Columbia University Press, 1998).

Condé, Maryse, 'Entretien de Maryse Condé avec Williams Sassine', *Recherche, Pedagogie et Culture*, 49 (1980), 64–6.

Connor, Steven, *The Book of Skin* (London: Reaktion, 2004).

Cooper, Frederick, *Colonialism in Question: Theory, Knowledge, History* (Berkeley and London: University of California Press, 2005).

Cose, Ellis, *Color-Blind: Seeing Beyond Race in a Race-Obsessed World* (New York: HarperCollins, 1997).

Cornaton, Michel, *Pouvoir et sexualité dans le roman africain* (Paris: L'Harmattan, 1990).

Coupland, Justine and Richard Gwyn, eds, *Discourse, the Body and Identity* (Basingstoke: Palgrave Macmillan, 2003).

Coussy, Denise, *La Littérature africaine moderne au sud du Sahara* (Paris: Karthala, 2000).

Coussy, Denise, and Jacques Chevrier, 'L'Errance chez Williams Sassine et V.S. Naipaul', *Notre Librairie*, 155–6 (2004), 68–75.

Cross, William E., *Shades of Black* (Philadelphia: Temple University Press, 1991).

Danielson, Dan, and Karen Engle, eds, *After Identity: A Reader* (London: Routledge, 1995).

Davidson, Hilda, ed., *Boundaries and Thresholds* (Stroud: Thimble Press, 1993).

Davis, L., *The Disability Studies Reader* (London: Routledge, 1997).
——, ed., *Enforcing Normalcy* (London: Verso, 1995).
De Blij, H.J., and Peter O. Muller, *Geography: Realms, Regions and Concepts* (London and New York: Wiley, 2003).
De Heusch, L., *Le Sacrifice dans les religions africaines* (Paris: Gallimard, 1986).
De Pina-Cabral, João, 'Albinos Don't Die: The Symbolic Ecology of Belief in Postcolonial Mozambique' (Unpublished paper, 2002).
Dehon, Claire L., *Le Réalisme africain: le roman francophone en Afrique subsaharienne* (Paris: L'Harmattan, 2002).
Deleuze, Gilles, *Nietzsche and Philosophy*. Trans. by Hugh Tomlinson (London: Continuum, 2006).
Devlieger, Patrick, 'The Logic of Killing Disabled Children: Infanticide', in *Disability and Social Exclusion: The Archaeology and Anthropology of Difference*, ed. by J. Hubert (London: Routledge, 2002), pp. 159–67.
——, 'Why Disabled? The Cultural Understanding of Physical Disability in an African Society' in *Disability and Culture*, ed. by Benedicte Ingstad and Susan Reynolds Whyte (Berkeley: University of California Press, 1995), pp. 94–104.
Diawara, Manthia, *In Search of Africa* (Cambridge, MA: Harvard University Press, 1998).
Dickinson, Daniel, 'Cancer stalks Tanzania's albinos'. BBC News Online, Dar es Salaam <http://news.bbc.co.uk/go/pr/fr/-/1/hi/world/africa/2982116.stm> [Accessed 13 January 2011].
Djatou, Médard, 'L'Albinos dans les représentations et pratiques culturelles des Ngante et Lengou de l'ouest Cameroun' (unpublished master's dissertation, University of Yaoundé I, 2001).
Donald, James, and Ali Rattansi, eds, *Race, Culture and Difference* (London: Sage, 1992).
Douglas, Mary, *Purity and Danger: An Analysis of Concepts of Pollution and Taboo* (London: Routledge, 1966).
——, *Implicit Meanings: Essays in Anthropology* (London: Routledge, 1975).
——, *Risk and Blame: Essays in Cultural Theory* (London: Routledge, 1992).
Dugast, Jacques, Irène Langlet et François Mouret, eds, *Littérature et interdits* (Rennes: Presses Universitaires de Rennes, 1998).
Dyer, Richard, *White: Essays on Race and Culture* (London: Routledge, 2004).
Edwards, Lee G., *Too White to be Black and too Black to be White: Living with Albinism* (Bloomington: Authorhouse, 2001).
Edwards, Rachel, *Myth and the Fiction of Michel Tournier and Patrick Grainville* (Lampeter: Edwin Mellen, 1996).
Elliott, Anthony, *Concepts of the Self* (Oxford: Blackwell, 2001).

Erny, Pierre, *L'Enfant et son mileu en Afrique noire* (Paris: L'Harmattan, 1987).
Ezeilo, B.N., 'Psychological Aspects of Albinism: an Exploratory Study with Nigerian (Igbo) Albino Subjects', *Social Science Medical Journal*, 29 (1989), 1129–31.
Fanon, Frantz, *Peau noire, masques blancs* (Paris: Editions du Seuil, 1972).
——, *Les Damnés de la terre* (Paris: Editions la découverte, 1987).
Featherstone, M., and B. Turner, eds, *Body and Society*, Volume 1 (London: Sage, 1995).
——, *Body and Society*, Volume 2 (London: Sage, 1996).
Featherstone, Mike, ed., *Body Modification* (London: Sage, 2000).
Fletcher, John, and Andrew Benjamin, eds, *Abjection, Melancholia and Love – The work of Julia Kristeva* (London: Routledge, 1990).
Forsdick, Charles, and David Murphy, eds, *Francophone Postcolonial Studies: A Critical Introduction* (London: Arnold, 2003).
Frank, A.W., *The Wounded Storyteller: Body, Illness and Ethics* (Chicago: University of Chicago Press, 1996).
Frankenberg, Ruth, ed., *Displacing Whiteness: Essays in Social and Cultural Criticism* (London: Duke University Press, 1997).
——, *White Woman, Race Matters: The Social Construction of Whiteness* (Minneapolis: University of Minnesota Press, 1993).
Fredrickson, George M., *Racism: A Short History* (Princeton: Princeton University Press, 2002).
Frosh, Stephen, *Identity Crisis: Modernity, Psychoanalysis and the Self* (London: Macmillan, 1991).
Gadjigo, Samba, *Ecole blanche, Afrique noire* (Paris: L'Harmattan, 1982).
Gaigher, R.J., P.M. Lund and E. Makuya, 'A Sociological Study of Children with Albinism at a Special School in the Limpopo Province', *Curationis*, 25 (2002), 4–11.
Gandhi, Leela, *Postcolonial Theory: A Critical Introduction* (New York: Columbia University, 1998).
Garnier, Xavier, *La Magie dans le roman africaine* (Paris: Presses universitaires de France, 1999).
Garog-Karady, Veronika, *Noirs et blancs. Leur image dans la littérature orale africaine* (Paris: SELAF, 1976).
Gascoigne, David, 'Patrick Grainville' in *Beyond the Nouveau Roman: Essays on the Contemporary French Novel* ed. by Michael Tilby (New York: 1990) 229–55.
Gates, Henry Louis, *'Race', Writing and Difference* (London: University of Chicago Press, 1992).
George, Rose, 'Beyond the Pale' *The Sunday Telegraph Magazine*, 5 October 2003.
Germain, Sylvie, *La Chanson des mal-aimants* (Paris: Gallimard, 2002).

Gibson, Nigel, *Rethinking Fanon: The Continuing Dialogue* (New York: Humanity Books, 1999).
Giguet, Frédéric, 'La construction tragique de l'identité dans l'œuvre romanesque de Williams Sassine' in Dominique Laporte (ed.), *L'autre en mémoire* (Presses Université Laval, 2006). Unpaginated.
Gilman, Sander L., *Difference and Pathology: Stereotypes of Sexuality, Race and Madness* (Ithaca and London: Cornell University Press, 1985).
Gilroy, Paul, *'There Ain't No Black in the Union Jack': The Cultural Politics of Race and Nation* (London: Hutchinson, 1987).
Ginsberg, Elaine K., ed., *Passing and the Fictions of Identity* (Durham: Duke University Press, 1996).
Girard, René, *Le Bouc émissaire* (Paris: Grasset, 1982).
Goffman, Erving, *Stigma – Notes on the Management of Spoiled Identity* (Harmondsworth: Penguin, 1963).
Goldberg, David Theo, and Ato Quayson, eds, *Relocating Postcolonialism* (London: Blackwell, 2002).
Gordon, Lewis R., T. Denean Sharpley-Whiting and Renee T. White, eds, *Fanon: A Critical Reader* (London: Blackwell, 1996).
Grenaud, F., *Et l'homme devint jaguar* (Paris: L'Harmattan, 1982).
Groce, N.E., 'Disability in Cross-Cultural Perspectives: Rethinking Disability', *Lancet*, 354 (1999), 756–7.
Grosz, Elizabeth, *Volatile Bodies: Toward a Corporeal Feminism* (Bloomington and Indianapolis: Indiana University Press, 1994).
Guidotti, R., 'Redefining Beauty', *LIFE Magazine* (1998) 65–9.
Guiounneau-Sinclair, F., 'El albinismo entro los Amérindios de Panama'. *Scienta: révista de investigacion de la Universidad de Panama*, 4.2 (1989), 41–50.
Hall, Stuart, 'Cultural Identity and Diaspora' in *Colonial Discourse & Postcolonial Theory: A Reader*, ed. by Patrick Williams and Laura Chrisman (London: Harvester Wheatsheaf, 1993), pp. 392–403.
——, 'Who Needs Identity?' in *The Identity Reader*, ed. by Paul du Gay, Jessica Evans and Peter Redman (London: Sage, 2000), pp. 15–31.
——, and Paul du Gay, *Questions of Cultural Identity* (London: Sage, 1996).
Hanquart-Turner, Evelyne, ed., *L'Hybridité* (Ivry-sur-Seine: Editions A3, 2001).
Hanson, Ben, *Takadini* (Zimbabwe: East Africa Education Publishers, 1997).
Hare, Robert, *Without Conscience: The Disturbing World of the Psychopaths Among Us* (New York: Guilford, 1999).
Harrison, Nicholas, *Postcolonial Criticism* (Cambridge: Polity Press, 2003).
Harrow, K., *Thresholds of Change in African Literature: The Emergence of a Tradition* (Portsmouth: Heinemann, 1994).

Hastings, Adrian, *Wirriyamu* (London: Search Press, 1974).
Hazoume, Flore, *La Vengeance de l'albinos* (Abidjan: EDILIS, 1996).
Hellum-Braathen, Stine, and Benedicte Ingstad, 'Albinism in Malawi: Knowledge and Belief from an African setting', *Disability and Society*, 21 (2006), 599–611.
Hilton-Barber, B., 'The Shadow People', *Marie Claire South Africa* (December 1997) 20–4.
Hitchcott, Nicki, *Women Writers in Francophone Africa* (Oxford: Berg, 2000).
——, and Laila Ibnlfassi, eds, *African Francophone Writing: A Critical Introduction* (Oxford: Berg, 1996).
Hogan, Patrick, *The Culture of Conformism: Understanding Social Consent* (Durham: Duke University Press, 2001).
Holloway, Judith, *Changing the Subject: Psychology, Social Regulation and Subjectivity* (London: Routledge, 1998).
Hong, E., H. Zeeb and M. Repacholi, 'Albinism in Africa as a Public Health Issue', *BMC Public Health*, 6 (2006), 212.
hooks, bell, *Feminist Theory: From Margin to Centre* (Boston: South End Press, 1984).
——, 'marginality as site of resistance' in *Out There: Marginalization and Contemporary Cultures* ed. by Russell Ferguson, Martha Gever, Trinh T. Minh-ha and Cornel West (New York: MIP, 1990), 341–3.
Howson, Alexandra, 'The Body in Consumer Culture' in *The Body in Society: An Introduction* (Cambridge: Polity Press, 2004).
Huggan, Graham, *The Postcolonial Exotic: Marketing the Margins* (London, Routledge: 2001).
Hunt, Paul, ed., *Stigma: The Experience of Disability* (London: Geoffrey Chapman, 1966).
Hutton, Margaret-Anne, 'Cultural Métissage: Victor Hugo, Egon Schiele and the Egyptian in Patrick Grainville's *Les Anges et les faucons*' in *Text(e)/image* ed. by Margaret-Anne Hutton (Durham: University of Durham, 1999), 176–90.
Ingstad, Benedicte, 'Coping Behaviour of Disabled Persons and their Families: Cross-Cultural Perspectives', *International Journal of Rehabilitation Research*, 11 (1988), 351–9.
——, and Susan Reynolds Whyte, *Disability and Culture* (Berkeley: University of California Press, 1995).
Jablonski, Nina G., *Skin: A Natural History* (Berkeley: University of California Press, 2006).
Jackson, Rosemary, *Fantasy: The Literature of Subversion* (London: Routledge, 2001).

Jacquard, Albert, *Éloge de la différence: la génétique et les hommes* (Paris: Seuil, 1978).

Jayne, Edward, *Negative Poetics* (Iowa City: University of Iowa Press, 1992).

Jeambrun, Pascale, 'L'Albinisme oculocutané: mises au point clinique, historique et anthropologique', *Archives de Pédiatrie*, 5.8 (1998), 896–907.

——, and Bernard Sergent, *Les Enfants de la lune: l'albinisme chez les Amérindiens* (Paris: Editions Inserm, 1991).

Johnson, Barbara, *The Feminist Difference – Literature, Psychoanalysis, Race and Gender* (London: Harvard University Press, 1998).

Kagore, F., and Patricia Lund, 'Oculocutaneous Albinism among Schoolchildren in Harare, Zimbabwe', *Journal of Genetic Medicine*, 32 (1995), 859–61.

Kanneh, Kadiatu, *African Identities: Race, Nation and Culture in Ethnography. Pan-Africanism and Black Literatures* (London: Routledge, 1998).

Kearney, Richard, *Strangers, Gods and Monsters: Interpreting Otherness* (London: Routledge, 2003).

Keita, Mamadi, *Revolt and its Expressions in the Works of Williams Sassine* (unpublished doctoral dissertation, University of Maryland, 2009).

Keith, Michael, *Place and Identity* (London: Routledge, 1993).

Kennedy, Randall, *Nigger: The Strange Career of a Troublesome Word* (New York: Vintage, 2002).

Kohn, Marek, *The Race Gallery: The Return of Racial Science* (London: Vintage, 1995).

Korpela, K.M., 'Place Identity as a Product of Environmental Self-Regulation', *Journal of Environmental Psychology*, 9 (1989), 241–56.

Krepps, David, *Cyborgism, Cyborgs, Performance and Society* (London: Lulu.com, 2007).

Kristeva, Julia, 'Interview' in *Julia Kristeva: Live Theory*, ed. by J. Lechte and M. Margaroni (London: Continuum, 2004).

——, *Pouvoirs de l'horreur: essai sur l'abjection* (Paris: Broché, 1980).

Kromberg, Jennifer, 'Albinism in the South African Negro: IV. Attitudes and the Death Myth', *Birth Defects*, 28 (1992), 159–66.

——, 'The Response of Black Mothers to the Birth of an Albino Child', *American Journal of Diseases of Children*, 21 (1987), 455–61.

——, D. Castle, E.M. Zwane and T. Jenkins, 'Albinism and Skin Cancer in Southern Africa', *Clinical Genetics*, 36 (1989), 43–52.

——, and T. Jenkins, 'Prevalence of Albinism in the South African Negro', *South African Medical Journal*, 61 (1982), 382–6.

Laburthe-Tolra, Philippe, *Initiations et sociétés secrètes au Cameroun: Essai sur la religion Beti* (Paris: Karthala, 1985).

Lacapra, Dominick, ed., *The Bounds of Race – Perspectives on Hegemony and Resistance* (Ithaca and London: Cornell University Press, 1991).
Lamming, George, *In the Castle of my Skin* (Ann Arbor: University of Michigan Press, 1953).
Lazarus, Neil, *Resistance in Postcolonial African Fiction* (New Haven: Yale University Press, 1990).
Le Breton, David, *Anthropologie du corps et modernité* (Paris: Presses Universitaires de France, 1992).
——, *La Sociologie du corps* (Paris: Presses Universitaires de France, 1992).
Leary, M.R., ed., *Interpersonal Rejection* (Oxford: Oxford University Press, 2001).
Lebon, Cécile, 'Review of Williams Sassine's *Mémoire d'une peau*', *Notre Librairie*, 136 (1999), 150–1.
Leder, Drew, *The Absent Body* (Chicago: University of Chicago Press, 1990).
Lévi-Strauss, Claude, *L'Identité* (Paris: Editions Grasset, 1977).
Lewis, Shireen K., *Race, Culture and Identity: Francophone West African and Caribbean Literature and Theory from Négritude to Créolité* (Oxford: Lexington, 2006).
Linton, Simi, *Claiming Disability: Knowledge and Identity* (New York: New York University Press, 1998).
Little, Roger, *Between Totem and Taboo: Black Man, White Woman in Francographic Literature* (Exeter: Exeter University Press, 2001).
——, *Nègres blancs: Représentations de l'autre autre* (Paris: L'Harmattan, 1995).
Lively, Adam, *Masks: Blackness, Race and the Imagination* (London: Vintage, 1999).
Lookingbill, D.P., G.L. Lookingbill and B. Leppard, 'Acintic Damage and Skin Cancer in Albinos in Northern Tanzania: Findings in 164 Patients Enrolled in an Outreach Skin Care Program', *Journal of the American Academy of Dermatology*, 32 (2006), 653–8.
Luande, J., C. Henschke and N. Mohammed, 'The Tanzanian Human Albino Skin: Natural History', *Cancer*, 55 (1985), 1823–8.
Lucky, A.W., 'Pigmentocracy Abnormalities in Genetic Disorders'. *Dermatologic Clinics*, 6.2 (1988), 193–203.
Lund, Patricia, 'Distribution of Oculocutaneous Albinism in Zimbabwe', *Journal of Medical Genetics*, 33 (1996), 641–4.
——, 'Health and Education of Children with Albinism in Zimbabwe', *Health Educational Research*, 16 (2001), 1–7.
——, 'Living with Albinism: A Study of Affected Adults in Zimbabwe', *Journal of Social Biology and Human Affairs*, 63 (1998), 3–10.

——, T.G. Maluleke, I. Gaigher and R. Gaigher, 'Variations in the Frequency of Albinism among Clans in the Venda Region of South Africa', *Journal of Medical Genetics*, 40 (2003), 823–38.

——, N. Puri, D. Durham-Pierre, R.A. King and M.H. Brilliant, 'Oculocutaneous Albinism in an Isolated Tonga Community in Zimbabwe', *Journal of Medical Genetics*, 34 (1997), 733–5.

Mamdani, Mahmood, *Citizen and Subject: Contemporary Africa and the Legacy of Late Colonialism* (Princeton: Princeton University Press, 1996).

Manning, Patrick, *Francophone Sub-Saharan Africa 1880–1995* (Cambridge: Cambridge University Press, 1995)

Marcato, Franca Falzoni, ed., *La Deriva della Francofonie: Figures et fantasmes de la violence dans les littératures francophones de l'Afrique subsaharienne et des Antilles* (Bologna: CLUEB, 1991).

Martin, Charles, *The White African American Body* (New Jersey: Rutgers, 2002).

Masha, Maryceline, 'What Kind of Black are You?' *The Tanzania Guardian* <http://www.vso.org.uk/publications/orbit/71/community.htm> [Accessed 30 June 2009].

Mbembe, Achille, 'Désordres, résistances et productivité', *Politique Africaine*, 39 (1991), 7–24.

——, *On the Postcolony* (Berkeley: University of California Press, 2001).

McBride, S., and B.J. Leppard, 'Attitudes and Beliefs of an Albino Population towards Sun Avoidance: Advice and Services provided by an Outreach Albino Clinic in Tanzania', *Archives of Dermatology*, 138 (2002), 629–32.

McClintock, Anne, 'The Angel of Progress: Pitfalls of the Term "Postcolonialism"' in *Colonial Discourse/ Postcolonial Theory*, ed. by F. Barker et al. (Manchester: Manchester University Press, 1994), pp. 252–66.

McNeil, Ronald, 'Black, Yet White: A Hated Color in Zimbabwe', *The New York Times* (9 February 1997).

Meier, August, *Along the Color Line: Explorations in the Black Experience* (Champaign: University of Illinois Press, 2003).

Mellor, Phillip A. and Chris Shilling, *Reforming the Body: Religion, Community and Modernity* (London: Sage, 1997).

Merleau-Ponty, Maurice, *Phenomenology of Perception*, trans. by Colin Smith (New York: Humanities Press, 1962).

Mihamlé, J.D., et H. Yonkeu, 'Les Albinos victimes des préjugés' *Ana-Bia Supplement*, 368 (1999) <http://www.peacelink.it/ana-bia/nr368/leo4.html>.

Milbury-Steen, Sarah L., *European and African Stereotypes in Twentieth-Century Fiction* (London: Macmillan, 1980).

Mikangou, Lyne, 'Les Albinos s'insurgent contre leur marginalisation: Témoignage de Ibouna, Joséphine' <http://www.genespoir.org/temoignage.htm>.
Mitchell, David, and Sharon Snyder, eds, *The Body and Physical Difference* (Ann Arbor: University of Michigan Press, 1997).
Mohanty, Chandra, *Feminism without Borders: Decolonizing Theory, Practicing Solidarity* (Durham: Duke University Press, 2003).
Moorcock, Michael, *The White Wolf's Son: The Albino Underground* (New York: Warner Aspect, 2005).
Moore-Gilbert, Bart, *Postcolonial Theory: Contexts, Practices, Politics* (London: Verso, 1997).
Morrison, Toni, *Playing in the Dark – Whiteness and the Literary Imagination* (London: Pan Books, 1993).
Morley, David, and Kuan-Hsing Chen, eds, *Stuart Hall: Critical Dialogues in Cultural Studies* (London: Routledge, 1996).
Mullard, Chris, *Race, Power and Resistance* (London: Routledge, 1985).
Murdoch, H. Adlai, and Anne Donadey, eds, *Postcolonial Theory and Francophone Literary Studies* (Gainesville: University Press of Florida, 2004).
Murphy, David, 'De-centring French Studies: Towards a Postcolonial Theory of Francophone Cultures', *French Cultural Studies*, 13.2 (2002), 165–85.
——, and Aedín Ní Loingsigh, eds, *Thresholds of Otherness/Autrement Mêmes: Identity and Alterity in French-Language Literatures* (London: Grant and Cutler, 2002).
Murphy, Robert, *The Body Silent: The Different World of the Disabled* (New York: Norton & Company Inc., 1990).
——, 'Encounters: The Body Silent in America' in *Disability and Culture* ed. by B. Ingstad and S.R. Whyte (New York: Henry Holt, 1995), 140–58.
Nachbar, Jack, and Kevin Lause, *Popular Culture: An Introductory Text* (Bowling Green, Ohio: Popular Press, 1992).
Naipaul, V.S. *The Writer and the World: Essays* (London: Picador, 2002).
Nakayama, Thomas K., and Judith N. Martin, eds, *Whiteness – The Communication of Social Identity* (London: Sage, 1998).
Nandjui, Pierre, *Houphouët-Boigny: L'Homme de la France en Afrique* (Paris: L'Harmattan, 1995).
Nederveen-Pieterse, Jan, *White on Black: Images of Africa and Blacks in Western Popular Culture* (New Haven, CT: Yale University Press, 1992).
Nietzsche, Friedrich, *The Will to Power as Art*, trans. by David Farrell Krell (San Francisco: HarperCollins, 1991).
Ngandu Nkashama, Pius, *Écrire à l'infinitif: la déraison de l'écriture dans les romans de Williams Sassine* (Paris: L'Harmattan, 2006).

Ngate, Jonathan, *Francophone African Fiction: Reading a Literary Tradition* (Trenton, NJ: Africa World Press, 1988).
Ngizi, Mongezi, *Black or White, Does it Matter?: My Journey with Albinism* (Pietermaritzburg: Lammergeyer, 2006).
Noonan, Harold, *Personal Identity* (London: Routledge, 1989).
Nooter, Mary H., ed., *La Notion de personne en Afrique noire* (Paris: CNRS, 1973).
Nyatetū-Waigwa, Wangarī, *The Liminal Novel: Studies in the Francophone-African Novel as Bildungsroman* (New York: Peter Lang, 1996).
Ogrizek, Marija, 'Les Albinos, enfants surnaturels des sirènes: approche ethnomédicale de l'albinisme en Afrique centrale', *Bulletin Ethnomédicale* (1983) 368–92.
——, 'Mami Wata: La sirène du Marigot', *Bulletin Ethnomédicale*, 44 (1984), 20–4.
Okulicz, J.F., R.S. Shah, R.A. Achwartz and C.K. Janniger, 'Oculocutaneous Albinism', *Journal of the European Academy of Dermatology and Venereology*, 17 (2003), 251–6.
Olson, Gary A., and Lynn Worsham, *Race, Rhetoric and the Postcolonial* (New York: State University of New York Press, 1999).
Onoja, Rose, and Andrew Airahuobhor, 'Albinos: Tales of Mockery, Rejection – Special Report', *Newswatch* (18 December 2006), 49–55.
——, 'Stop It! Albinos are not "Unfortunate Europeans": Interview with Jake Epelle, President of Albino Foundation', *Newswatch* (18 December 2006), 50–7.
Ortonne, J.P., 'Piebaldism, Wardenburg's Syndrome and Related Disorders', *Dermatologic Clinics*, 6.2 (1988), 205–16.
Osborne, Peter, and Stella Sandford, *Philosophies of Race and Ethnicity* (London: Continuum, 2002).
Pakenham, Thomas, *The Scramble for Africa: The White Man's Conquest of the Dark Continent from 1876–1912* (New York: Avon, 1991).
Page, Robert M., *Stigma* (London: Routledge, 1984).
Parent Ugochukwu, Françoise, 'The Devil's Colours: A Comparative Study of French and Nigerian Folktales', *Oral Tradition*, 21.2 (2007), 1–18.
Parry, Albert, *Tattoo: Secrets of a Strange Art* (New York: Dover Publications, 2006).
Parry, Benita, 'Resistance Theory/Theorising Resistance or Two Cheers for Nativism', in *Colonial Discourse/Postcolonial Theory*, ed. by F. Barker, Hulme and M. Inversen (Manchester: Manchester University Press, 1994) 172–96.
Petit, Susan, '*Le Tyran éternel* by Patrick Grainville', *French Review*, 73 (1999), 163–4.
Pickering, Michael, *Stereotyping–The Politics of Representation* (Basingstoke: Palgrave, 2001).

Pile, Steve, and Michael Keith, eds, *Geographies of Resistance* (London: Routledge, 1997).
Pitts, Victoria L., *In the Flesh: The Cultural Politics of Body Modification* (New York: Palgrave Macmillan, 2003).
Pobi-Asamani, Kwadwo O., *W.E.B. Du Bois. His Contributions to Pan-Africanism* (San Bernadino: Borgo Press, 1994).
Pothier, Anne, and Richard Devlin, *Critical Disability Theory: Essays in Philosophy, Politics, Policy and Law* (Vancouver: UBC Press, 2006).
Punday, Daniel, *Narrative Bodies* (Basingstoke: Palgrave Macmillan, 2003).
Quashie, Kevin Everod, *Black Women, Identity, and Cultural Theory: (Un)Becoming the Subject* (New Brunswick, NJ: Rutgers University Press, 2004).
Quayson, Ato, and David Goldberg, eds, *Relocating Postcolonialism* (Oxford: Blackwell, 2002).
Reichl, Susanne, and Mark Stein, eds, *Cheeky Fictions: Laughter and the Postcolonial* (Amsterdam: Rodopi, 2005).
Ricœur, Paul, *Oneself as Another* (Chicago: University of Chicago Press, 1992).
Reif-Hulser, Monika, *Borderlands: Negotiating Boundaries in Post-Colonial Writing* (Atlanta: Rodopi, 1999).
Roediger, David R., *Colored White: Transcending the Racial Past* (Berkeley: University of California Press, 2003).
Rosello, Mireille, *Declining the Stereotype: Ethnicity and Representation in French Cultures* (Dartmouth: University of New England Press, 1997).
Roseneil, Sasha, and Julie Seymour, eds, *Practising Identities: Power and Resistance* (Basingstoke: Macmillan, 1999).
Roth, Philip, *The Human Stain* (London: Vintage, 2001).
Roy, Archie W., and Robin Spinks, *Real Lives: Personal and Photographic Perspectives on Albinism* (Glasgow: Albinism Fellowship, 2005).
Roy, Namba, *Black Albino* (London: Longman African Writers, 1988).
Russell, Kathy, *The Colour Complex: The Politics of Skin Colour among African Americans* (London: Harcourt Brace Janovich, 1993).
Said, Edward, *Culture and Imperialism* (London: Vintage, 1994).
——, *Orientalism* (London: Penguin, 1995).
Saint-André Utudjan, Eliane, 'Le Thème de la folie dans la littérature africaine contemporaine', *Présence Africaine*, 115 (1980), 118–47.
Salomé, Lou, *Nietzsche* (Champaign: University of Illinois Press, 2001).
Sanchez, Maria Carla, and Linda Schlossberg, eds, *Passing and the Fictions of Identity* (Durham: Duke University Press, 1996).
Sargisson, Lucy, *Utopian Bodies and the Politics of Transgression* (London: Routledge, 2000).

Schembri, Michèle, 'Liberté, égalité, minorité' *Images*, 41 (1999), 9–10.
Schuerkens, Ulrike, *La Colonisation dans la littérature africaine* (Paris: L'Harmattan, 1994).
Schipper, Mineke, *Imagining Insiders: Africa and the Question of Belonging* (London: Cassell, 1999).
Scott, James C., *Domination and the Arts of Resistance: Hidden Transcripts* (London: Yale University Press, 1990).
——, *Weapons of the Weak: Everyday forms of Peasant Resistance* (New Haven: Yale University Press, 1985).
Sebestyén, György, *A Man Too White* (Riverside, CA: Ariadne Press, 1993).
Segal, Ronald, *The Black Diaspora* (London: Faber & Faber, 1995).
Sergent, B., 'Les Trois excellentes raisons de se débarrasser de ce bébé-là', *Nouvelle Revue d'Ethnopsychiatre*, 12 (1988), 11–54.
Serres, Michel, *Les cinq sens* (Paris: Grasset, 1998).
Sharp, Joanne P., Paul Routledge, Chris Philo and Ronan Paddison, eds, *Entanglements of Power: Geographies of Domination and Resistance* (London: Routledge, 2000).
Sheers, Owen, *The Dust Diaries* (London: Faber and Faber, 2004).
Shildrick, Margrit, *Embodying the Monster: Encounters with the Vulnerable Self* (London: Sage, 2002).
Shilling, Chris, *The Body and Social Theory* (London: Sage, 1993).
Shirazi, Fageheh, *The Veil Unveiled: The Hijab in Modern Culture* (Gainesville: Florida University Press, 2003).
Sloane, William, *The Craft of Writing* (New York: W.W. Norton & Co. Ltd, 1979).
Small, V.A., 'Sociological Studies of People of Colour with Albinism' (1998) <http://www.zebracorn.com>.
Smith, Robert P. Jr., 'The Political Voice of African Youth in Williams Sassine's *Le Jeune homme de sable*', *College Language Association Journal*, 37 (1994), 316–27.
Sneider, Sharon L., and David T. Mitchell, *Cultural Locations of Disability* (Chicago: University of Chicago Press, 2006).
Sollors, Werner, *Neither Black nor White, yet Both: Thematic Explorations of Interracial Literature* (New York: Oxford University Press, 1997).
Solomon, Robert C., *In the Spirit of Hegel: A Study of G.W.F. Hegel's Phenomenology of Spirit* (New York: Oxford University Press, 1983).
Sontag, Susan, *Illness as Metaphor* (New York: Random House, 1977).
Sow, Alioune, 'Forbidden Bodies: Relocation and Empowerment in Williams Sassine's novels', *Matatu Journal for African Culture and Society*, 29 (2005), 207–20.
Soyinka, Wole, *Myth, Literature and the African World* (Cambridge: Cambridge University Press, 1976).

Spivak, Gayatri Chakravorty, 'Acting Bits/Identity Talk', *Critical Enquiry* 18.4 (1992), 770–803.
Stangor, Charles, *Stereotypes and Prejudice: Essential Readings* (London: Psychology Press, 2002).
Stafford, Andy, 'Review of H. Adlai Murdoch and Anne Donadey (eds), *Postcolonial Theory and Francophone Literary Studies*', *French Studies*, 61.1 (2007), 124–5.
Stewart, Susan, *On Longing: Narratives of the Miniature, the Gigantic, the Souvenir, the Collection* (Durham: Duke University Press, 1993).
Stiker, Henri-Jacques, *Corps infirmes et sociétés* (Paris: Aubier Montaigne, 1982).
Sundquist, Eric J., ed., *New Essays on Uncle Tom's Cabin* (Cambridge: Cambridge University Press, 1993).
Synott, A., *The Body Social: Symbolism, Self and Society* (London: Routledge, 1993).
Syrotinski, Michael, *Singular Performances: Reinscribing the Subject in Francophone African Writing* (London: University of Virginia Press, 2002).
Thomson, Rosemary Garland, ed., *Freakery: Cultural Spectacles of the Extraordinary Body* (New York: New York University Press, 1996).
——, *Extraordinary Bodies: Figuring Physical Disability in American Culture and Literature* (Chicago: University of Chicago Press, 1997).
Toffoletti, Kim, *Cyborgs and Barbie Dolls: Feminism, Popular Culture and the Post-human Body* (London: I.B. Tauris & Co., 2007).
Tromsness-Mitchell, Elizabeth, *Albinism in the Family* (Bloomington: Authorhouse, 2004).
Turner, Bryan, *The Body and Society* (Oxford: Blackwell, 1984).
Turner, Victor, *The Ritual Process* (New York: Aldine de Gruyter, 1969).
TuSmith, Bonnie, 'The Inscrutable Albino in Contemporary Ethnic Literature', *Amerasia Journal*, 19.3 (1993), 85–102.
Ugbolue, A., *Parental Perceptions and Roles in the Socialization of the Albino Child* (Los Angeles: University of California Press, 1975).
Vander-Kolk, Charles J., 'Albinism: A Survey of Attitudes and Behaviour', *Journal of Visual Impairment and Blindness*, 1.2 (1983), 149–58.
Van Gennep, Arnold, *The Rites of Passage* (Chicago: University of Chicago Press, 1960).
Van Thomson, Carlyle, *The Tragic Black Buck: Racial Masquerading in the American Literary Imagination* (New York: Peter Lang, 2004).
Von Hippel, William, *The Social Outcast: Ostracism, Social Exclusion, Rejection, and Bullying* (New York: Taylor and Francis, 2005).
Wa Thiong'o, Ngũgĩ, *Decolonizing the Mind: The Politics of Language in African Literature* (London: James Curry, 1986).

Walker, Nancy, *A Very Serious Thing: Women's Humor and American Culture* (Minneapolis: University of Minnesota Press, 1988).

Wan, Nathalie, 'Orange in a World of Apples: The Voices of Albinism', *Disability and Society*, 18.3 (2003), 277–96.

Wendeler, Catherine, 'The Embodiment of Wrath in Two Postcolonial Prophecies: *La Vie et demie* by Sony Labou Tansi and *Mémoire d'une peau* by Williams Sassine', *Imperium*, 2 (2001), 380–91.

Werbner, Pnina, 'Essentialising Essentialism; Essentialising Silence: Ambivalence and Multiplicity in the Constructions of Racism and Ethnicity'. In P. Werbner and T. Modood, eds, *Debating Cultural Hybridity: Multicultural Identities and the Politics of Antiracsim* (London: Zed Books, 1997), 226–54.

——, 'The Limits of Cultural Hybridity: On Ritual Monsters, Poetic Licence and Contested Postcolonial Purifications', *Journal of the Royal Anthropological Institute*, 184 (2001), 133–52.

Werbner, Richard, and Terence Ranger, *Postcolonial Identities in Africa* (London: Zed Books, 1996).

Whatmore, Sarah, *Hybrid Geographies: Natures, Cultures, Spaces* (London: Sage, 2002).

Wideman, John Edgar, *Sent for You Yesterday* (Boston: Houghton Mifflin, 1997).

Wieviorka, Michel, *La Différence* (Paris: Editions Balland, 2001).

Williams, Kipling, *Ostracism: The Power of Silence* (New York: Guilford Press, 2002).

Williams, Patrick, and Laura Chrisman, eds, *Colonial Discourse and Postcolonial Theory: A Reader* (London: Harvester Wheatsheaf, 1993).

Woodward, Kathryn, ed., *Identity and Difference* (London: Sage, 1997).

Wylie, Hal, and Berndt Lindfors, *Multiculturalism and Hybridity in African Literatures* (Trenton: AWP, 2000).

Yakuba, A., and O.A. Mabogunje, 'Skin Cancer in African Albinos', *Acta Oncologia*, 32 (1993), 621–2.

Young, Robert J.C., *Colonial Desire: Hybridity in Theory, Culture and Race* (London: Routledge 1995).

——, *White Mythologies: Writing, History and the West* (London: Routledge, 1990).

Zinhumwe, T., 'Not Black Enough', *Inter Press Service* (26 November 1996).

Zola, Irving, *Missing Pieces: A Chronicle of Living with a Disability* (Philadelphia: Temple University Press, 1982).

Zylinska, Joanna, *The Cyborg Experiments: The Extensions of the Body in the Media Age* (London: Continuum, 2002).

Bibliography

Websites:

Albinism Fellowship UK <http://www.albinism.org.uk>.
Albinism in Popular Culture <http://www.lunaeterna.net/popcult>.
Albinism World Alliance <http://awa.albinism.org>.
The Albino Foundation in Nigeria <http://www.thealbinofoundation.com>.
Albinos sans frontières <http://www.asf-awb.org>.
Comptoir Littéraire <http://www.comptoirlitteraire>.
Genespoir <http://www.genespoir.org>.
International Albinism Centre <http://albinism.med.umn.edu>.
Le Temps du Monde <http://www.letemps.ch/tour/reportages/jour322.html>.
Low Vision Organisation <http://www.lowvision.org/albinism.htm>.
National Organisation for Albinism and Hypopigmentation (NOAH) <http://www.albinism.org>.
Positive Exposure <http://www.positiveexposure.org>.
Skinema <http://www.skinema.com>.
VSO <http://www.vso.org.uk/publications/orbit/71/community.htm>.
Who's Who in France <http://www.whoswho.fr>.
Zebracorn <http://www.zebracorn.com>.

Index

albinism 1
    discrimination 53
    genetics 15, 39
    HIV AIDS 67
    inscrutable albino 170
    language 2, 52, 54
    media representation 51
    misconceptions 65
    myth v, 57, 73, 74, 202, 206, 212
    nègre blanc 2
    ocular albinism 2
    oculocutaneous albinism 1
    prevalence 2
    stereotype v, 57, 58, 59, 62, 82, 211
Anzieu, Didier 36, 37, 198

Bakhtin, Mikhail 48
    grotesque 49
belonging 98
Berlin Conference 131
Bhabha, Homi 15, 16, 58, 113, 160
Blumenbach, Johann Friedrich 27
body, the 20, 49, 164
    albino body 23
    body modification 99
    colour 25
    inscription 166
    skin 24, 37
    tattooing 100
boundary, the 131, 139

centre/margin dichotomy 134

Destremau, Didier: *Nègre blanc* 4, 8, 25, 29, 30, 38, 43, 44, 45, 52, 55, 61, 62, 64, 65, 66, 68, 69, 70, 72, 75, 77, 78, 89, 90, 92, 99, 100, 102, 103, 108, 110, 114, 116, 121, 122, 126, 127, 128, 130, 132, 134, 137, 138, 139, 142, 145, 158, 159, 163, 182, 183, 193, 197
disability 20, 41, 42, 45, 55, 58, 62, 84, 88, 91, 118, 135, 171, 180, 183, 189
Douglas, Mary 118

exclusion 87, 91

Fanon, Frantz 3, 16, 17, 26, 32, 35, 50, 53, 102, 124, 143, 144, 151, 157, 158, 160, 172, 173, 184, 199, 200, 203, 204
    Les Damnés de la terre 17, 124, 203
    Peau noire, masques blancs 3, 16, 17, 26, 32, 35, 50, 53, 102, 143, 144, 151, 157, 158, 172, 184, 203
forest 122
freakery 51
    freak shows 51, 128

Grainville, Patrick: *Le Tyran Èternel* 4, 5, 8, 16, 25, 38, 45, 46, 61, 66, 68, 69, 75, 79, 80, 99, 100, 109, 114, 115, 116, 121, 122, 123, 124, 139, 142, 145, 160, 161, 163, 182, 183, 185, 186, 193, 197

Hanson, Ben: *Takadini* 10, 38, 40, 43, 52, 66, 68, 78, 193, 204

Hegel, Georg Wilhelm Friedrich 151
humour 150, 152, 153, 155

identity 105, 126, 137, 138, 141, 169, 171, 179
    malleability of 105
    multiple identities 106
    theories of 172
inclusion 103
interstitial space 114

Keita, Salif 109, 160
Kristeva, Julia 119

lactification 33, 102
Linnaeus, Carl 26

madness 8, 49, 71, 75, 176
marginality 133
margins 115
masks 154
Merleau-Ponty, Maurice 32
métissage 97, 175
misrecognition 108
mission civilisatrice 33
myth 128

passing 95
postcolonialism
    critique 18
    theory 17, 18, 115, 189
Postcolonialism 15
    Francophone postcolonial studies 18
power 141, 163
    and resistance 149, 152
    and violence 142, 146, 148
Prichard, James Cowles 29

race 3, 26
    blackness 28, 46
    chromatic ambivalence 31, 134, 186
    whiteness 28, 30
Roy, Namba: *Black Albino* 10, 40, 52, 115, 120, 194, 211

sacrifice 77
Said, Edward 15, 16
Sassine, Williams
    Mémoire d'une peau 4, 6, 7, 8, 9, 10, 22, 31, 32, 39, 44, 47, 49, 52, 53, 54, 63, 71, 75, 82, 95, 97, 101, 105, 106, 114, 119, 121, 122, 125, 135, 141, 142, 146, 147, 148, 149, 152, 154, 155, 156, 158, 159, 160, 161, 164, 165, 167, 169, 170, 174, 176, 178, 182, 183, 184, 187, 188, 194, 197, 198, 207
    Wirriyamu 4, 6, 7, 8, 9, 31, 33, 34, 48, 49, 52, 54, 60, 64, 69, 76, 78, 79, 80, 81, 89, 90, 107, 110, 111, 114, 115, 117, 120, 121, 122, 125, 135, 136, 137, 139, 142, 143, 144, 174, 176, 177, 178, 182, 183, 187, 188, 194, 197, 198, 204
scapegoating 81
Serres, Michel 25
skin
    skin cancer 44
    social canvas 47
social exile 93
stigmatisation 30, 57, 69, 70, 71, 72, 84, 160

threat 116

visibility 1

Wideman, John Edgar: *Sent For You Yesterday* 32

Modern French Identities
Edited by Peter Collier

This series aims to publish monographs, editions or collections of papers based on recent research into modern French Literature. It welcomes contributions from academics, researchers and writers in British and Irish universities in particular.

Modern French Identities focuses on the French and Francophone writing of the twentieth century, whose formal experiments and revisions of genre have combined to create an entirely new set of literary forms, from the thematic autobiographies of Michel Leiris and Bernard Noël to the magic realism of French Caribbean writers.

The idea that identities are constructed rather than found, and that the self is an area to explore rather than a given pretext, runs through much of modern French literature, from Proust, Gide and Apollinaire to Kristeva, Barthes, Duras, Germain and Roubaud.

This series reflects a concern to explore the turn-of-the-century turmoil in ideas and values that is expressed in the works of theorists like Lacan, Irigaray and Bourdieu and to follow through the impact of current ideologies such as feminism and postmodernism on the literary and cultural interpretation and presentation of the self, whether in terms of psychoanalytic theory, gender, autobiography, cinema, fiction and poetry, or in newer forms like performance art.

The series publishes studies of individual authors and artists, comparative studies, and interdisciplinary projects, including those where art and cinema intersect with literature.

Volume 1   Victoria Best & Peter Collier (eds): Powerful Bodies.
            Performance in French Cultural Studies.
            220 pages. 1999. ISBN 3-906762-56-4 / US-ISBN 0-8204-4239-9

Volume 2   Julia Waters: Intersexual Rivalry.
            A 'Reading in Pairs' of Marguerite Duras and Alain Robbe-Grillet.
            228 pages. 2000. ISBN 3-906763-74-9 / US-ISBN 0-8204-4626-2

Volume 3	Sarah Cooper: Relating to Queer Theory. Rereading Sexual Self-Definition with Irigaray, Kristeva, Wittig and Cixous. 231 pages. 2000. ISBN 3-906764-46-X / US-ISBN 0-8204-4636-X
Volume 4	Julia Prest & Hannah Thompson (eds): Corporeal Practices. (Re)figuring the Body in French Studies. 166 pages. 2000. ISBN 3-906764-53-2 / US-ISBN 0-8204-4639-4
Volume 5	Victoria Best: Critical Subjectivities. Identity and Narrative in the Work of Colette and Marguerite Duras. 243 pages. 2000. ISBN 3-906763-89-7 / US-ISBN 0-8204-4631-9
Volume 6	David Houston Jones: The Body Abject: Self and Text in Jean Genet and Samuel Beckett. 213 pages. 2000. ISBN 3-906765-07-5 / US-ISBN 0-8204-5058-8
Volume 7	Robin MacKenzie: The Unconscious in Proust's *A la recherche du temps perdu*. 270 pages. 2000. ISBN 3-906758-38-9 / US-ISBN 0-8204-5070-7
Volume 8	Rosemary Chapman: Siting the Quebec Novel. The Representation of Space in Francophone Writing in Quebec. 282 pages. 2000. ISBN 3-906758-85-0 / US-ISBN 0-8204-5090-1
Volume 9	Gill Rye: Reading for Change. Interactions between Text Identity in Contemporary French Women's Writing (Baroche, Cixous, Constant). 223 pages. 2001. ISBN 3-906765-97-0 / US-ISBN 0-8204-5315-3
Volume 10	Jonathan Paul Murphy: Proust's Art. Painting, Sculpture and Writing in *A la recherche du temps perdu*. 248 pages. 2001. ISBN 3-906766-17-9 / US-ISBN 0-8204-5319-6
Volume 11	Julia Dobson: Hélène Cixous and the Theatre. The Scene of Writing. 166 pages. 2002. ISBN 3-906766-20-9 / US-ISBN 0-8204-5322-6
Volume 12	Emily Butterworth & Kathryn Robson (eds): Shifting Borders. Theory and Identity in French Literature. VIII + 208 pages. 2001. ISBN 3-906766-86-1 / US-ISBN 0-8204-5602-0
Volume 13	Victoria Korzeniowska: The Heroine as Social Redeemer in the Plays of Jean Giraudoux. 144 pages. 2001. ISBN 3-906766-92-6 / US-ISBN 0-8204-5608-X

Volume 14   Kay Chadwick: Alphonse de Châteaubriant:
             Catholic Collaborator.
             327 pages. 2002. ISBN 3-906766-94-2 / US-ISBN 0-8204-5610-1

Volume 15   Nina Bastin: Queneau's Fictional Worlds.
             291 pages. 2002. ISBN 3-906768-32-5 / US-ISBN 0-8204-5620-9

Volume 16   Sarah Fishwick: The Body in the Work of Simone de Beauvoir.
             284 pages. 2002. ISBN 3-906768-33-3 / US-ISBN 0-8204-5621-7

Volume 17   Simon Kemp & Libby Saxton (eds): Seeing Things.
             Vision, Perception and Interpretation in French Studies.
             287 pages. 2002. ISBN 3-906768-46-5 / US-ISBN 0-8204-5858-9

Volume 18   Kamal Salhi (ed.): French in and out of France.
             Language Policies, Intercultural Antagonisms and Dialogue.
             487 pages. 2002. ISBN 3-906768-47-3 / US-ISBN 0-8204-5859-7

Volume 19   Genevieve Shepherd: Simone de Beauvoir's Fiction.
             A Psychoanalytic Rereading.
             262 pages. 2003. ISBN 3-906768-55-4 / US-ISBN 0-8204-5867-8

Volume 20   Lucille Cairns (ed.): Gay and Lesbian Cultures in France.
             290 pages. 2002. ISBN 3-906769-66-6 / US-ISBN 0-8204-5903-8

Volume 21   Wendy Goolcharan-Kumeta: My Mother, My Country.
             Reconstructing the Female Self in Guadeloupean Women's Writing.
             236 pages. 2003. ISBN 3-906769-76-3 / US-ISBN 0-8204-5913-5

Volume 22   Patricia O'Flaherty: Henry de Montherlant (1895–1972).
             A Philosophy of Failure.
             256 pages. 2003. ISBN 3-03910-013-0 / US-ISBN 0-8204-6282-9

Volume 23   Katherine Ashley (ed.): Prix Goncourt, 1903–2003: essais critiques.
             205 pages. 2004. ISBN 3-03910-018-1 / US-ISBN 0-8204-6287-X

Volume 24   Julia Horn & Lynsey Russell-Watts (eds): Possessions.
             Essays in French Literature, Cinema and Theory.
             223 pages. 2003. ISBN 3-03910-005-X / US-ISBN 0-8204-5924-0

Volume 25   Steve Wharton: Screening Reality.
             French Documentary Film during the German Occupation.
             252 pages. 2006. ISBN 3-03910-066-1 / US-ISBN 0-8204-6882-7

Volume 26   Frédéric Royall (ed.): Contemporary French Cultures and Societies.
             421 pages. 2004. ISBN 3-03910-074-2 / US-ISBN 0-8204-6890-8

Volume 27   Tom Genrich: Authentic Fictions.
             Cosmopolitan Writing of the Troisième République, 1908–1940.
             288 pages. 2004. ISBN 3-03910-285-0 / US-ISBN 0-8204-7212-3

Volume 28 Maeve Conrick & Vera Regan: French in Canada.
Language Issues.
186 pages. 2007. ISBN 978-3-03-910142-9

Volume 29 Kathryn Banks & Joseph Harris (eds): Exposure.
Revealing Bodies, Unveiling Representations.
194 pages. 2004. ISBN 3-03910-163-3 / US-ISBN 0-8204-6973-4

Volume 30 Emma Gilby & Katja Haustein (eds): Space.
New Dimensions in French Studies.
169 pages. 2005. ISBN 3-03910-178-1 / US-ISBN 0-8204-6988-2

Volume 31 Rachel Killick (ed.): Uncertain Relations.
Some Configurations of the 'Third Space' in Francophone Writings
of the Americas and of Europe.
258 pages. 2005. ISBN 3-03910-189-7 / US-ISBN 0-8204-6999-8

Volume 32 Sarah F. Donachie & Kim Harrison (eds): Love and Sexuality.
New Approaches in French Studies.
194 pages. 2005. ISBN 3-03910-249-4 / US-ISBN 0-8204-7178-X

Volume 33 Michaël Abecassis: The Representation of Parisian Speech in
the Cinema of the 1930s.
409 pages. 2005. ISBN 3-03910-260-5 / US-ISBN 0-8204-7189-5

Volume 34 Benedict O'Donohoe: Sartre's Theatre: Acts for Life.
301 pages. 2005. ISBN 3-03910-250-X / US-ISBN 0-8204-7207-7

Volume 35 Moya Longstaffe: The Fiction of Albert Camus. A Complex Simplicity.
300 pages. 2007. ISBN 3-03910-304-0 / US-ISBN 0-8204-7229-8

Volume 36 Arnaud Beaujeu: Matière et lumière dans le théâtre de Samuel Beckett:
Autour des notions de trivialité, de spiritualité et d'« autre-là ».
377 pages. 2010. ISBN 978-3-0343-0206-8

Volume 37 Shirley Ann Jordan: Contemporary French Women's Writing:
Women's Visions, Women's Voices, Women's Lives.
308 pages. 2005. ISBN 3-03910-315-6 / US-ISBN 0-8204-7240-9

Volume 38 Neil Foxlee: Albert Camus's 'The New Mediterranean Culture':
A Text and its Contexts.
349 pages. 2010. ISBN 978-3-0343-0207-4

Volume 39 Michael O'Dwyer & Michèle Raclot: Le Journal de Julien Green:
Miroir d'une âme, miroir d'un siècle.
289 pages. 2005. ISBN 3-03910-319-9

Volume 40 Thomas Baldwin: The Material Object in the Work of Marcel Proust.
188 pages. 2005. ISBN 3-03910-323-7 / US-ISBN 0-8204-7247-6

Volume 41	Charles Forsdick & Andrew Stafford (eds): The Modern Essay in French: Genre, Sociology, Performance. 296 pages. 2005. ISBN 3-03910-514-0 / US-ISBN 0-8204-7520-3
Volume 42	Peter Dunwoodie: Francophone Writing in Transition. Algeria 1900–1945. 339 pages. 2005. ISBN 3-03910-294-X / US-ISBN 0-8204-7220-4
Volume 43	Emma Webb (ed.): Marie Cardinal: New Perspectives. 260 pages. 2006. ISBN 3-03910-544-2 / US-ISBN 0-8204-7547-5
Volume 44	Jérôme Game (ed.): Porous Boundaries : Texts and Images in Twentieth-Century French Culture. 164 pages. 2007. ISBN 978-3-03910-568-7
Volume 45	David Gascoigne: The Games of Fiction: Georges Perec and Modern French Ludic Narrative. 327 pages. 2006. ISBN 3-03910-697-X / US-ISBN 0-8204-7962-4
Volume 46	Derek O'Regan: Postcolonial Echoes and Evocations: The Intertextual Appeal of Maryse Condé. 329 pages. 2006. ISBN 3-03910-578-7
Volume 47	Jennifer Hatte: La langue secrète de Jean Cocteau: la *mythologie personnelle* du poète et l'histoire cachée des *Enfants terribles*. 332 pages. 2007. ISBN 978-3-03910-707-0
Volume 48	Loraine Day: Writing Shame and Desire: The Work of Annie Ernaux. 315 pages. 2007. ISBN 978-3-03910-275-4
Volume 49-50	Forthcoming.
Volume 51	Isabelle McNeill & Bradley Stephens (eds): Transmissions: Essays in French Literature, Thought and Cinema. 221 pages. 2007. ISBN 978-3-03910-734-6
Volume 52	Marie-Christine Lala: Georges Bataille, Poète du réel. 178 pages. 2010. ISBN 978-3-03910-738-4
Volume 53	Patrick Crowley: Pierre Michon: The Afterlife of Names. 242 pages. 2007. ISBN 978-3-03910-744-5
Volume 54	Nicole Thatcher & Ethel Tolansky (eds): Six Authors in Captivity. Literary Responses to the Occupation of France during World War II. 205 pages. 2006. ISBN 3-03910-520-5 / US-ISBN 0-8204-7526-2
Volume 55	Catherine Dousteyssier-Khoze & Floriane Place-Verghnes (eds): Poétiques de la parodie et du pastiche de 1850 à nos jours. 361 pages. 2006. ISBN 3-03910-743-7
Volume 56	Forthcoming.

Volume 57　Helen Vassallo: Jeanne Hyvrard, Wounded Witness:
The Body Politic and the Illness Narrative.
243 pages. 2007. ISBN 978-3-03911-017-9

Volume 58　Marie-Claire Barnet, Eric Robertson and Nigel Saint (eds):
Robert Desnos. Surrealism in the Twenty-First Century.
390 pages. 2006. ISBN 3-03911-019-5

Volume 59　Michael O'Dwyer (ed.): Julien Green, Diariste et Essayiste.
259 pages. 2007. ISBN 978-3-03911-016-2

Volume 60　Kate Marsh: Fictions of 1947: Representations of Indian
Decolonization 1919–1962.
238 pages. 2007. ISBN 978-3-03911-033-9

Volume 61　Lucy Bolton, Gerri Kimber, Ann Lewis and Michael Seabrook (eds):
Framed! : Essays in French Studies.
235 pages. 2007. ISBN 978-3-03911-043-8

Volume 62　Lorna Milne and Mary Orr (eds): Narratives of French Modernity:
Themes, Forms and Metamorphoses. Essays in Honour of David
Gascoigne.
365 pages. 2011. ISBN 978-3-03911-051-3

Volume 63　Ann Kennedy Smith: Painted Poetry: Colour in Baudelaire's
Art Criticism.
253 pages. 2011. ISBN 978-3-03911-094-0

Volume 64　Sam Coombes: The Early Sartre and Marxism.
330 pages. 2008. ISBN 978-3-03911-115-2

Volume 65-66 Forthcoming.

Volume 67　Alison S. Fell (ed.): French and francophone women facing war /
Les femmes face à la guerre.
301 pages. 2009. ISBN 978-3-03911-332-3

Volume 68　Elizabeth Lindley and Laura McMahon (eds):
Rhythms: Essays in French Literature, Thought and Culture.
238 pages. 2008. ISBN 978-3-03911-349-1

Volume 69　Georgina Evans and Adam Kay (eds): Threat: Essays in French
Literature, Thought and Visual Culture.
248 pages. 2010. ISBN 978-3-03911-357-6

Volume 70　John McCann: Michel Houellebecq: Author of our Times.
229 pages. 2010. ISBN 978-3-03911-373-6

Volume 71　Jenny Murray: Remembering the (Post)Colonial Self:
Memory and Identity in the Novels of Assia Djebar.
258 pages. 2008. ISBN 978-3-03911-367-5

| Volume 72 | Susan Bainbrigge: Culture and Identity in Belgian Francophone Writing: Dialogue, Diversity and Displacement. 230 pages. 2009. ISBN 978-3-03911-382-8 |

Volume 73-74 Forthcoming.

| Volume 75 | Elodie Laügt: L'Orient du signe: Rêves et dérives chez Victor Segalen, Henri Michaux et Emile Cioran. 242 pages. 2008. ISBN 978-3-03911-402-3 |

| Volume 76 | Suzanne Dow: Madness in Twentieth-Century French Women's Writing: Leduc, Duras, Beauvoir, Cardinal, Hyvrard. 217 pages. 2009. ISBN 978-3-03911-540-2 |

| Volume 77 | Myriem El Maïzi: Marguerite Duras ou l'écriture du devenir. 228 pages. 2009. ISBN 978-3-03911-561-7 |

| Volume 78 | Forthcoming. |

| Volume 79 | Jenny Chamarette and Jennifer Higgins (eds): Guilt and Shame: Essays in French Literature, Thought and Visual Culture. 231 pages. 2010. ISBN 978-3-03911-563-1 |

| Volume 80 | Vera Regan and Caitríona Ní Chasaide (eds): Language Practices and Identity Construction by Multilingual Speakers of French L2: The Acquisition of Sociostylistic Variation. 189 pages. 2010. ISBN 978-3-03911-569-3 |

| Volume 81 | Margaret-Anne Hutton (ed.): Redefining the Real: The Fantastic in Contemporary French and Francophone Women's Writing. 294 pages. 2009. ISBN 978-3-03911-567-9 |

| Volume 82 | Elise Hugueny-Léger: Annie Ernaux, une poétique de la transgression. 269 pages. 2009. ISBN 978-3-03911-833-5 |

| Volume 83 | Peter Collier, Anna Magdalena Elsner and Olga Smith (eds): Anamnesia: Private and Public Memory in Modern French Culture. 359 pages. 2009. ISBN 978-3-03911-846-5 |

| Volume 84 | Adam Watt (ed./éd.): Le Temps retrouvé Eighty Years After/80 ans après: Critical Essays/Essais critiques. 349 pages. 2009. ISBN 978-3-03911-843-4 |

| Volume 85 | Louise Hardwick (ed.): New Approaches to Crime in French Literature, Culture and Film. 237 pages. 2009. ISBN 978-3-03911-850-2 |

| Volume 86 | Forthcoming. |

Volume 87 Amaleena Damlé and Aurélie L'Hostis (eds): The Beautiful and the Monstrous: Essays in French Literature, Thought and Culture.
237 pages. 2010. ISBN 978-3-03911-900-4

Volume 88 Alistair Rolls (ed.): Mostly French: French (in) Detective Fiction.
212 pages. 2009. ISBN 978-3-03911-957-8

Volume 89 Bérénice Bonhomme: Claude Simon : une écriture en cinéma.
359 pages. 2010. ISBN 978-3-03911-983-7

Volume 90 Barbara Lebrun and Jill Lovecy (eds): *Une et divisible?* Plural Identities in Modern France.
258 pages. 2010. ISBN 978-3-0343-0123-7

Volume 91 Pierre-Alexis Mével & Helen Tattam (eds): Language and its Contexts/ Le Langage et ses contextes: Transposition and Transformation of Meaning?/ Transposition et transformation du sens ?
272 pages. 2010. ISBN 978-3-0343-0128-2

Volume 92 Forthcoming.

Volume 93 Michaël Abecassis et Gudrun Ledegen (éds): Les Voix des Français Volume 1: à travers l'histoire, l'école et la presse.
372 pages. 2010. ISBN 978-3-0343-0170-1

Volume 94 Michaël Abecassis et Gudrun Ledegen (éds): Les Voix des Français Volume 2: en parlant, en écrivant.
481 pages. 2010. ISBN 978-3-0343-0171-8

Volume 95 Forthcoming.

Volume 96 Charlotte Baker: Enduring Negativity: Representations of Albinism in the Novels of Didier Destremau, Patrick Grainville and Williams Sassine.
226 pages. 2011. ISBN ISBN 978-3-0343-0179-4

Volume 97 Florian Grandena and Cristina Johnston (eds): New Queer Images: Representations of Homosexualities in Contemporary Francophone Visual Cultures.
246 pages. 2011. ISBN 978-3-0343-0182-4

Volume 98 Florian Grandena and Cristina Johnston (eds): Cinematic Queerness: Gay and Lesbian Hypervisibility in Contemporary Francophone Feature Films.
354 pages. 2011. ISBN 978-3-0343-0183-1